January 2020

Hold On, Let Go

Many blessings!

love

Nadine Arundt

Library and Archives Canada Cataloguing in Publication

Sands, Nadine, 1968-, author
    Hold on, let go : facing ALS with courage and hope / Nadine Sands.

Issued in print and electronic formats.
ISBN 978-1-77141-101-1 (pbk.).--ISBN 978-1-77141-102-8 (html)

    1. Sands, Michael, 1962- --Health 2. Sands, Nadine, 1968-.
3. Amyotrophic lateral sclerosis--Patients--Canada--Biography.
4. Amyotrophic lateral sclerosis--Patients--Family relationships--
Canada. I. Title.

RC406.A24S25 2015   362.1'968390092   C2014-907750-5
                                            C2014-907751-3

Hold On, Let Go

Facing ALS with Courage and Hope

Nadine Sands with Michael Sands

First Published in Canada 2015 by Influence Publishing

Book Cover Design: Trista Baldwin
Editor: Nina Shoroplova
Assistant Editor: Susan Kehoe
Production Editor: Jennifer Kaleta
Typeset: Greg Salisbury
Portrait & Cover Photographer: Amanda Waschuk

Citations

For

Erin, Nathan, Madison,

Leah,

Michaela, Luke,

the Georges and Sheilas of our lives,

our big sisters,

and

our big brothers.

Testimonials

"In her book, Nadine pulls back the veil of her family's experience with ALS, enough to give us a taste of the emotions, the practical challenges, the needed support, and necessary encouragement that are required to navigate these treacherous waters. This book offers lessons in both how to handle life with purpose and enjoyment, as well as lessons for facing an impending death with grace and dignity. Be prepared to have your eyes opened and your heart touched."
Dr. Tom Blackaby, Author, International Speaker, Blackaby Ministries International

"As athletes we talk about making every minute count and never giving up. Nadine and Mike, along with their family, are true inspirations with their approach and attitude towards life. With ALS recently impacting one of my loved ones, I find Nadine and Mike's commitment to hope, faith, and love incredibly uplifting and moving"
Carla MacLeod, Two-Time Olympic Gold Medalist, Canadian National Women's Hockey Team

"In my position as the Executive Director of the ALS Society of BC, I am motivated every day by the courage of the people we serve. Nadine and Mike are an amazing couple who are an inspiration to everyone they meet. ALS cannot take away the incredible love they have for each other."
Wendy Toyer, Executive Director, ALS Society of BC

Acknowledgements

A big thank you to everyone who helped me make this dream a reality, including the following:

The brilliant team at Influence Publishing—Julie, Nina, Sue, Trista, Gulnar, and Alina—thanks for your patience, wisdom, insight, and understanding. You're amazing; I'm grateful!

Thanks to my dear friend Adele who said after my first blog post, "You are going to write a book someday, and I will come with you to your book signings."

Thanks also to the other friends who encouraged me to write a book, including the grandma of one of Madison's former hockey teammates. She had no idea that her message, "I read your blog ... it's inspiring! You should publish your posts someday," and other kind words, came at the exact moment I was wrestling with the beginnings of *Hold On, Let Go*. I had just closed my laptop in frustration and discouragement, thinking "forget it," when I received this thoughtful and timely message. That was a turning point for me and I never looked back.

To my sounding board—Aunty Vicki, Carol, Elanna, my Mom and Dad, Craig, Pauline, Aunty M, and Brad and Karen W—thanks for your feedback, your encouragement, and your votes of confidence.

My Mom and Dad have always assumed I could do anything; that definitely helped me do this. Their constant support and prayers have been invaluable.

Erin, thank you for your endless encouragement; Nathan, for your strength and support; and Madison for your salads, sandwiches, gluten-free muffins, and other help.

My sister Elanna has kept me going and has stood beside me

all the way. She inspires me every day. Thanks to her and her family for their continual help and support.

To other sisters, Pat and Aileen, and Mum Sheila for all your care, for being there for us and for making this journey easier to tread.

Mike, who has been so patient with me throughout this process and supportive as always—thanks for your smiles; each one motivates me to keep going and to keep looking up. You are my hero … my superman!

Mike's caregivers, you are incredible—you are such a blessing to us.

To my blog readers—thanks for reading and thanks for caring.

God, who is my Rock, my strength, my everything—without You I am nothing. Mike and I both agree, we are absolutely nothing without You!

Contents

Prologue

Fried Chicken Bucket List—September 18, 2011— by Mike Sands

I always considered anyone who dies before fifty as dying "young." Anyone who dies between fifty and sixty is "early." Anyone between sixty and seventy has had "a full life." Anyone seventy and above has lived "a long life."

In a few months I'll be turning fifty and I now have a sense of relief; "Whew, I made it to fifty ..." even though it's still young. (Meanwhile all the other people hitting fifty are dreading it.)

It's funny how your fear of things disappears when someone tells you that you don't have long to live. My fear of flying is no longer a problem. Who needs sunscreen anymore? Using aluminum pots may cause Alzheimer's; I say bring on the scrambled eggs.

It's ironic that I have always kept an eye on being physically fit. I generally eat the right foods, I've never smoked, and I exercise regularly; all that and I'm still left with this diagnosis. All these years of staying healthy, I could have been eating tasty fried chicken and French fries every day. I guess I have some catching up to do.

I've never been afraid of dying. I've heard too many good things about heaven. I think we all have trepidation about dying as God puts the fear of dying in us so that we don't jump off a cliff in our teens after getting jilted for the first time. If we instinctively knew there was a better life waiting for us, we wouldn't cherish and hang on to this life. I think we're supposed to live a good productive life while leaving our mark and making a difference in the lives of the people around us. This can be accomplished without necessarily living a long life; as Abe Lincoln says, "It's not the years in your life that count; it's the life in your years."

When I was given this terminal diagnosis, the thought raced through my head that I have to do the things that I've always wanted to do but didn't get around to. Climb Mount Everest? Never had the inclination. Go to Hawaii? Not on my bucket list. See the Eiffel tower? A postcard will do. I was at a loss to find something that I had missed out on. I do believe I have experienced everything that I wanted to experience. It doesn't look like I'm going to live until I'm sixty or seventy, but I'm happy to have lived "a full life."

I have to go now, my Kentucky Fried Chicken order has just arrived. What's this? They forgot the gravy!

Introduction

Faith, hope, and love—these things remain and are what we hold on to as we learn to let go ...

My husband Mike and I have become very familiar with letting go since Mike was diagnosed in March 2011 with the terminal illness, ALS (Amyotrophic Lateral Sclerosis), also known as Lou Gehrig's disease.

Mike was a very active, athletic man working two jobs as a registered nurse. He stopped working the day of diagnosis and began his quest to fight the effects of ALS. He made dramatic changes to his diet and exercise routine among other things, but his strongest ammunition already existed within himself: an unwavering faith, a very positive attitude, a wonderful sense of humour, and courage; and that is what inspired me to start my blog, called *ALS With Courage.*

My blog was a great way to keep friends and family informed of Mike's constantly changing condition and it was also a great way to reveal his incredible spirit.

In the beginning, I thought it was simply an inspiring story about a courageous man and his ALS, but it quickly became so much more than that. It became a collection of lessons for me, including the lesson of letting go.

Mike has let go of working, walking, talking, eating, moving, and slowly he lets go of breathing. And I am letting go of him. Together we have had to let go of the wonderful life we built, a life we knew and loved. But what we thought was the best wasn't, and what we have now is better, and that's what my blog has revealed to me. With each loss, we gain; by losing so much, we have more than we could imagine. And throughout, we give God the praise and rely more and more on Him.

Every blog post has been like a piece of a puzzle ... gently placed in my hand one at a time. A big beautiful picture is being pieced together slowly—a corner piece here, a middle piece there. It's like a Monet under construction right before my eyes, in big childlike puzzle pieces.

We all have a picture being pieced together, and this one is ours ...

Chapter 1
Trust Rock

They say that behind every good man is a great woman. I say, behind me is an exceptional man. This is one reason why ...

Mike is a really smart guy, but you wouldn't know it to see him or even when you first meet him. I learned he was smart over time. I would hear him speaking with other people and think, "Wow, how do you know that?" He was so unassuming and he always spoke to people at their level. It quickly became apparent that Mike is way smarter than I am, but I never feel dumb around him. In fact, he always makes me feel smarter and more capable than I am.

Years ago, well before ALS, I told Mike I was going to write something someday. He believed it more than I did. Even though I wasn't a writer and he was actually a very good one, and even though I had never displayed any writing qualities, he believed it because he believed in me. He never doubted me. He has always encouraged and supported me. I feel like a flower in a well-watered garden.

Little did I know at the time I told Mike I was going to be a writer someday that he would become my reason to write. And the following excerpts from my blog is the "something" I wrote.

It's an ongoing story of my hero and the-forever-changed me.

The Journey of Courage Begins—September 1, 2011

"Courageous" is not a word I would have used to describe my husband Mike until recently. Not that he has ever given me any reason to believe he isn't courageous, but there are just so many other words I would have used first to describe him, such as funny, intelligent, handsome, silly, positive, hardworking, loving, generous, kind, and trustworthy. Even though "courageous" isn't in the top ten, he has displayed courage many times throughout our twenty-three years of marriage.

Mike exhibited plenty of courage when he decided to go back to school to become a registered nurse. He was just a few credits away from receiving his degree in Political Science with a minor in History and decided to change direction and go into nursing. He didn't necessarily have a desire to become a nurse but rather, he felt called. With our first two children still in diapers, Mike obeyed the call and went right back to square one. He juggled the books in the day and a job at night and found time in between to help me raise the kids. Now that took some courage!

Oxford dictionary describes courage as "strength in the face of pain or grief." That sounds about right. On March 7, 2011, "courage" moved up to the top ten.

We did our research and suspected Mike had ALS before he was diagnosed. We were really hoping it was MS or Parkinson's disease or anything else, but on that cool, sunny afternoon, Mike was diagnosed with ALS.

Later that same day Mike said, "Everyone in history has died and that's a fact! It's such a good thing to know where you are going when you do." In shock, he was finding comfort that if the diagnosis was right, and ALS soon takes his life, he has a home in heaven.

We read from the Book of James in the Bible, "Blessed is the one who perseveres under trial because, having stood the test, that person will receive the crown of life that the Lord has promised to those who love Him," James 1:12[1]

And so, Mike began his journey of courage ... and hope!

---

[1]Unless otherwise stated, all Bible quotes are from the New International Version.

What Is ALS Anyway?—September 3, 2011

I didn't really know what ALS was. I knew it was a debilitating
and terminal disease, so I knew it wasn't good. Life expectancy is
two to five years from the onset of symptoms. Mike experienced
his first symptom—muscle fasciculation (muscle twitching)—a
little over a year ago. He didn't think much of it. Working two
jobs, he was overworked and under-rested. He just brushed off
the twitch and carried on. He's not the type to worry. It was
when he noticed a loss of strength in his right hand and some
muscle atrophy in the same hand and forearm that he became
a little worried. After some research on the internet, and a visit
to our chiropractor who expressed concern, he realized it could
be serious, so he finally went to the doctor who referred him
to a neurologist, who delivered the bad news. Mike stopped
working, caught up on some much needed rest, changed his
diet, and noticed some improvements. So, when he went for a
second opinion, he was extremely hopeful. This doctor surely
would say a mistake was made and he would be fine … not! A
third and fourth opinion confirmed the same diagnosis—ALS.

ALS stands for Amyotrophic Lateral Sclerosis. It is a fatal,
progressive neurological condition that results in the paralysis
of voluntary muscles and loss of the ability to mobilize,
swallow, speak, and eventually, to breathe.

The cause is unknown, although just last week there were
reports in the news that the cause could relate to a build-up of
protein in the nerves in the brain and spinal column. Hopefully
this finding expedites the process of finding a cure.

Mike remained hopeful for a misdiagnosis even after seeing
four different doctors. He said something about how God was

practising medicine when those guys were still in diapers.

Hope is something we cling to … a misdiagnosis, a miraculous healing, a cure … any of the above will do. But even more than hope, we cling to the God who provides the hope, and trust Him to determine Mike's future.

"Be joyful in hope, patient in affliction, faithful in prayer."
Romans 12:12

In one of my favourite books, *My Utmost for His Highest*, the author Oswald Chambers writes: "Fill your mind with the thought that God is there. And once your mind is truly filled with that thought, when you experience difficulties it will be as easy as breathing for you to remember, 'My heavenly Father knows all about this!'"

You Don't Know What You've Got till It's Gone— September 4, 2011

A dear friend was on my mind this morning when I woke up. Karen was diagnosed with breast cancer recently and had a mastectomy two days ago. An email from a friend said that Karen was doing well, eating cinnamon buns and cracking jokes about her hospital roommates. The email went on to say that a group of Karen's visitors squeezed into the washroom to view the newly vacant space on Karen's chest. One day a woman has two breasts and the next day, she has one. It made me think how we don't always appreciate something until it's gone.

Two weeks after Mike's diagnosis, as I pondered my appreciation for him and the threat he might soon be gone,

I wrote in my journal the following: "Mike does my income taxes ... he pays the bills ... he makes most of the money. He washes the kitchen floor ... and the inside of the microwave ... he picks up the dog pooh in the backyard ... he gets the oil changed in the car ... he helps the kids with homework. He turns off the hockey game so I can watch the end of the show, *Love It or List It* ... he holds my hand when I know he wants to let go ... he makes me laugh ... he tells me I'm beautiful. He never expects dinner, but appreciates it when there is some ... he never complains ... he is patient, forgiving, thoughtful. I really appreciate him and can't imagine my life without him."

"Let us be grateful to people who make us happy; they are
the charming gardeners who make our souls blossom."
Marcel Proust

Look Away, I'm Hideous—September 5, 2011

I came home from the gym the other day to find Mike on our bed with a towel over his head and blood on his knees and hands. I knew he had fallen off his bike because Madison, our younger daughter, had called Erin, our older daughter (who was with me at the gym), to tell us the news. Mike told Madison not to call, but she was so upset she didn't know what else to do. Erin and I hurried home.

Mike was a little choked up and I could tell more damage had been done on the inside than on the outside. He told me what happened—he was going too fast around a corner so he put the brakes on hard. He has lost most of the use of his right hand, so he put the brake on hard with his left hand, which is the front brake, which caused the bike to throw him over the handlebars, placing him face first on the cement.

I could hear the discouragement in his voice from under the towel. This is a man who has been an athlete all his life. Someone who could, at one time, run a 35-minute 10K (10 kilometres). Who could, up until a few months ago, run a 6-minute mile, and was a strong competitor on the soccer field.

I knew what Mike was thinking under that towel. He was thinking that perhaps he had taken his bike for its last spin ... perhaps ALS has taken away his ability to ride a bike, like it's taken away his ability to run and play soccer.

I assured Mike the accident could have happened to anyone. I told him about the time I did the very same thing. I was a teenager, on my way to a softball game. I can still see myself being propelled over my handlebars, landing smack dab on the side walk ... like it happened in slow motion. I showed up to my game with a bloody nose and a couple of fat lips.

We talked for a little while and soon Mike felt better. Back to his old self, he quoted Kramer from Seinfeld, and said, "Look away, I'm hideous," as he took the towel off his face and exposed the wounds. He assured me that the fall wouldn't keep him down and that he would be back on his bike in no time.

We watched our two-year-old granddaughter, Leah, that evening, and she and Mike compared "owies" on their knees.

That night, when Mike and I went to bed, I put more Polysporin® on his owies and he fell asleep. I couldn't help but stare at him while he slept. He looked so peaceful in spite of his wounds—a goose egg and big cut over his left eyebrow, a big bump and road rash under the same eye, scratches down his nose, and a big fat lip.

A few days later, when Mike's hands felt better, he got right back on his bike.

"Courage is never to let your actions be influenced by your fears."
Arthur Koestler

Trust Rock—September 7, 2011

Marked on our calendar for today is an appointment with the ALS Team at GF Strong Rehabilitation Hospital in Vancouver. There is a new drug for ALS that is still under trial and Mike was going to be a part of the study. We were excited about this new drug and were praying that Mike would get the real thing and not the placebo … turns out, he isn't getting either. Too many people signed up for the study, so some of them were scratched … Mike being one of them.

Mike got the call while I was out one day last week. He told me the news without any emotion. I couldn't believe it when he told me, as we had been gearing up for this for a long time. I had to call the doctor's office myself and hear about this grave injustice with my own ears. They told me what Mike told me and said they were sorry, but the study was closed. That train has left the station and we missed it. Mike said it was okay because this new drug isn't the cure anyway and he is waiting for the cure. At that moment, I heard the Lord in His quiet voice remind me that I trust in Him … that we trust God and believe He is in control. We have committed our lives to Him and have put all our faith in Him, so we weren't going to let this news shake that faith.

"Trust in the Lord with all your heart, and lean not on your own understanding; in all your ways submit to Him, and He will make your paths straight."
Proverbs 3:5-6

I received an email from Erin last night. It was her first day at UBC (University of British Columbia). She finished her Bachelor's degree at the University of the Fraser Valley in Abbotsford, BC (British Columbia) in December and lived at home while she waited for the teaching program at UBC to start. Mike and I moved her to Point Grey two days ago. She is going to be a French Immersion teacher. Anyway, she relayed all the happenings of the day in her witty way, making me laugh out loud, and ended the message with the following: "I have science class in the morning and the professor told us to bring something that describes science to us. I'm bringing the 'trust rock' you gave me [a rock with the word 'trust' on it], because I trust that the scientists of today will find a cure for ALS. I trust that God has created a brain out there that will find it! I am praying every single day!"

~ ~ ~ ~ ~ ~ ~

You could also say, "Trust the Rock!" as God is referred to as "the Rock" many times in the Bible.

"Trust in the Lord forever, for the Lord Himself is the Rock eternal."
Isaiah 26:4

Scar Face—September 12, 2011

Mike is very patient and patience is a virtue and that's a good thing. But here is an example where his patience goes too far. The wounds on his face from his bike accident have healed quickly. The only evidence the fall ever happened is a couple of ugly scabs on his face that he has been walking around with for the last week.

I've been trying to persuade him to let me take them off. "No way, I'll be scarred for life," he says.

The scabs were the size and texture of bran flakes. I told him to stay away from my bowl of cereal, because those scabs were hanging by a thread and I wasn't fond of the idea of one of them falling into my breakfast. Mike just laughed and said it was a good way of adding protein to my diet.

When the scabs turned a gross shade of green, I told him, "That's it, they're coming off!"

He just laughed and pushed me away. The point is Mike is very patient ... with scabs and almost everything else.

All joking aside, Mike is incredibly patient. While out grocery shopping, I often bump into someone I know and stop to chat. Mike waits patiently. When he comes with me clothes shopping, I eye up the dressing room, and he eyes up a comfortable seat ... and waits patiently. His response when I ask how something looks on me: "You would look good in a burlap sack!"

He could be starving and wait another three hours to eat ... he is good at waiting. Line-ups, construction, flight delays, burnt dinners, doctor's appointments … he'll wait.

Mike continues to exercise a lot of patience as he adapts to the changes in his life caused by ALS. It takes more time and more effort to do the things he used to do with ease. Getting dressed, brushing his teeth, fixing a snack, taking a shower, tying his shoes—all of these things are more difficult now. His speech is affected by the illness as well, so when he speaks, he goes slowly. He will repeat himself if something is unclear, or he will pause and smile while he waits for his lips and his brain to get on the same page.

Most of us less patient people would become very frustrated, even angry. But as I watch Mike, I learn. His wonderful example of patience is teaching me something about being more patient and I am humbled.

The Best Medicine—September 14, 2011

Mike is on medication for some symptoms of ALS. Before his diagnosis, he never took anything … he didn't have to, because he was never sick. In spite of the pill bottles lined up on our counter now, we still believe that laughter is the best medicine.

Mike likes getting a good laugh, whether it's making someone else laugh or himself. A while ago, when he told me to pick up a cigar for him while I was out, I knew he was up to something, because he doesn't smoke cigars. We recently replaced one of our toilets and when I got home with Mike's cigar, he had the old toilet set up in the backyard. He had me take his picture sitting on the toilet, reading a newspaper, smoking a cigar.

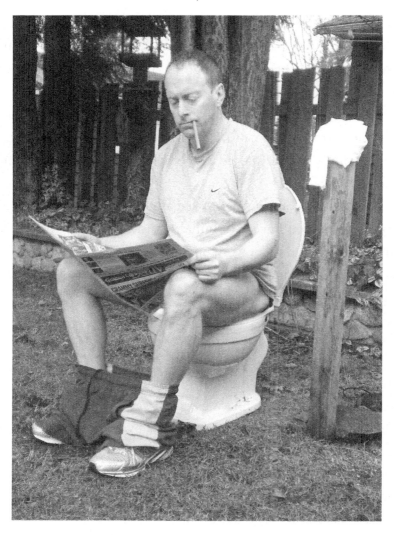

He is actually a bit of a prankster. It's pretty much routine for him to place a 50 kg bag of dog food in the middle of the aisle at the grocery store and watch people manoeuvre their buggies around it. I caught him teaching my friend Carol's two boys that trick one day when we were visiting them in Vernon, BC. Along with the pranks at the grocery store, the ice cream fight at the Dairy Queen, and writing in the snow with their pee at

Silver Star ski resort, it was a banner day for Levi and Max. Recalling the events of our time out together to their mom, the boys killed themselves laughing. Carol says Mike is like a celebrity around there.

Mike and I laugh a lot. Even more now because heightened emotions is a symptom of ALS, it's called "Pseudobulbar Affect." Once one of us gets started, the other joins in and there is no stopping us.

It's natural to become depressed after receiving bad news … like hearing you have a terminal illness. But, after the initial shock of our bad news wore off a little, Mike was up to his old tricks. Don't get me wrong, there are lots of tears as well, but the laughter far outweighs the grief.

Love Is Patient and Kind—September 16, 2011

The words "Love is patient, love is kind" are written on our bedroom wall. It's the first message I read in the morning and the last one I read at night. I try to live by that message, but of course, it's a challenge sometimes.

Mike and I have a good relationship. We can honestly say we are happily married. Of course it's not perfect … no marriage is. There are things that irritate me about him and I guess there are a few things that irritate him about me. We have just learned to accept each other's imperfections over the years.

Mike's table manners are terrible. He eats too fast; he is messy and noisy. But I knew that going in, so I try to ignore it. Sometimes I'll nudge him under the table if we are with other people.

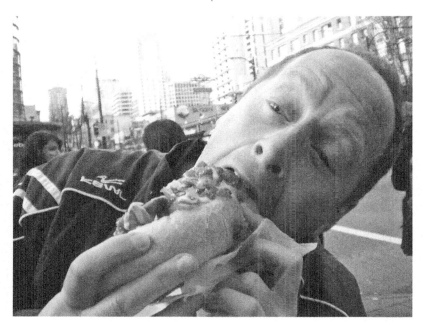

I'm not a good cook. In fact, I have burned many meals, dishcloths, oven mitts, even a phone once. Mike says, "It's okay, you can't be good in all the rooms," and happily eats whatever I serve.

I will admit though, I get very annoyed when Mike leaves wet towels on the bed, and he does it frequently. He has a habit of drying off after a shower and dropping his towel on my side of the bed while looking in his drawer for clean socks and underwear.

When I was sure Mike and I were going to grow old together, I didn't think twice about taking five or ten minutes to tell him off for leaving a wet towel on my side of the bed. But last night when Mike did it again, I quickly stopped myself when I got mad.

"I can't spare five or ten minutes to tell him off," I thought.

He looked at me with the wet towel in my hand and knowing what I was thinking, he said, "Yes, dear?"

There was a long pause and then we both broke out in laughter. We spent about five or ten minutes laughing and talking, and then we went to bed.

"Love is patient, love is kind. It does not envy, it does not boast, it is not proud. It does not dishonour others, it is not self-seeking, it is not easily angered, it keeps no record of wrongs. Love does not delight in evil but rejoices with the truth. It always protects, always trusts, always hopes, always perseveres."

I Corinthians 13:4-7

Ride Like the Wind—September 20, 2011

Mike had another incident on his bike the other day. Although concerning, this incident wasn't as serious as the last one. He had some trouble steering around a corner, over the sidewalk, and into the bike lane, and unfortunately was unable to stop his bike before riding into the side of a big black truck. Thankfully, the truck was almost at a stop as it was approaching a stop sign and no one was hurt. I should say no one was physically hurt … Mike's ego was a little crumpled.

I was riding behind him and saw the whole thing happen. I felt frustrated and sad for Mike as I watched him and the man driving the truck exchange a few words. Mike got upset and rightfully so. Just a few short months ago, he was working two jobs, bench-pressing 225 pounds, and able to leap tall buildings in a single bound, and now he is trying to explain to some insensitive guy in a black truck that he hadn't been drinking.

Anyway, I am now a little worried about Mike riding his bike on the busy roads in our neighbourhood.

Mike has hyperactive reflexes; he also experiences rigid movement, limited range of motion, and muscle weakness. But on his bike, he feels great. I'm a fitness instructor and I teach all types of fitness classes, including studio cycling (spinning), and I can't keep up with him; he rides like the wind. So needless to say, he is out on his bike every day. I go with him most of the time, but sometimes he goes alone.

Trying not to be obvious about my concern, the other day when he said he was going for a ride I insisted he wait for me, so I could go with him. He looked at me and said, "You want to come with me because you are worried about me, aren't you?"

I insisted I wasn't worried, and that I just wanted to be with him, which was true, but he was also right.

Since then, we have gone for a number of bike rides, and I have made sure I'm available to go along every time. He says, "You're just coming so you can catch me if I fall."

I want to go with him so I can save him from the evil traffic and the nasty sharp corners and the speeding cars and the drivers who aren't paying attention. I want to warn him of any hazards and, YES, catch him if he falls. The only problem is I am totally incapable of doing all those things. Not to mention, he has always been the one who protects me ... the one who catches me when I fall.

Soon after his diagnosis, Mike started to thank me in advance for taking care of him. I told him I knew he would do the same for me and I reminded him that we are a team.

Last night as I laid Mike's legs on my lap and massaged his

feet, I said a silent prayer. I prayed that as difficult as it gets, the Lord would enable me to do my best to take good care of the love of my life and number one teammate.

> *"Believers look up—take COURAGE!*
> *The angels are nearer than you think."*
> **Billy Graham**

Big Sisters—September 21, 2011

My sister Elanna called the other day to ask if we needed any cat food. She saw a great deal on "Friskies®" and thought of us ... or, I guess she thought of our cats.

My sister has been the best big sister a girl could have. She has looked out for me since day one. My parents tell me how when they brought me home from the hospital, Elanna had all the children in the neighbourhood there to welcome me. She doted on me then, and she dotes on me now. She encourages me, compliments me, brags about me, helps me, gives me things, and so on. She is like an extension of my parents who lavish me with love and gifts, and continue to take care of me even though I'm all grown up.

Mike is the youngest in his family as well. He has an older brother and three older sisters. Along with his parents, his siblings live in Toronto with their families. His sister Pat, all of eleven months older than Mike, said not long ago, "Michael will always be the baby."

During a recent visit, she definitely treated him like the kid brother he has always been to her. He was well taken care of ... meals and gifts, including a bunch of new socks and a new electric razor. Pretty much anything he needs, she has him covered. She even chased away some bullies ... or, maybe I'm getting that confused with Mike's childhood stories growing up in Highland Creek, Scarborough, Ontario in the 1960s.

Mike's sister Aileen made a surprise visit the weekend we participated in our first ALS walk in Abbotsford. Erin, who organized our team (the "I Like Mike" Team), tried to persuade her aunt Aileen to join us in the walk, but she kept coming up with "a bunch of lame excuses," as Erin put it.

Little did we know, she had booked her flight and was keeping the visit a secret. Just before we were going to start the walk, one of the event coordinators came up to Erin and told her there was an unexpected team member in the crowd. We looked around and there, to our surprise, was Aileen. When Mike saw Aileen, he hurried over to her and gave her a huge hug. Mike and his siblings aren't huggers, but this embrace was the real thing and we all were moved to tears.

Today, Mike received a card in the mail from his oldest sister Moira. On the front of the card it said, "No matter where you are ..." and on the inside it said, "You are here," with a picture of a bear holding his hand up against his heart.

We are well taken care of and extremely loved! We are so thankful for our big sisters!

So, to our big sisters ... No matter where you are, you are here (I am holding my hand against my heart).

~ ~ ~ ~ ~ ~ ~

When the idea to start *ALS With Courage* first came to me, I didn't question it. I thought it was the perfect thing to do … like I was called to do it. It became my mission to make sure family and friends could follow us on our new journey with terminal illness.

I didn't consider the disease a gift at the time, but journaling online about it was. I thought I was doing something for others, but I soon realized that God was doing something for me. He gave me this outlet for my benefit … to express my sorrow and joy, to learn incredible things about Him, and to slowly loosen my grip on my husband and on many things I hold tight.

The therapeutic value was and still is tremendous!

Chapter 2
Hold On ... Loosely

What I noticed right away when I first met my friend Carol and what I loved about her was her transparency. She was real and she wasn't afraid to show it. Unlike me, who tries hard to keep the ugly covered and the pretty prominent, Carol was open with who she is ... the good, the bad, and everything in-between. I was drawn to her realness—to her gutsy way of letting her true colours shine through. She didn't try to hide a past, or pretend everything was perfect. Her freedom in this area was beauty to me, and it drew me in.

Impressed but convicted, next to this window, I felt like a wall. Carol's transparency allowed the redemption power of God along with His light and love to shine through. Over the years, this transparency has inspired me to become more window, less wall ... though, that work is still under construction.

I consider my friendship with Carol a match made in heaven. We complement each other well; many of her strengths are my weaknesses and vice versa. It's an "Iron sharpens iron, and one person sharpens another" (Proverbs 27:17) friendship for sure.

Before Carol moved to Vernon, BC with her husband Scott and their boys in October 2010, she and I got together frequently to visit and to pray. Now, most of our communication is through emails. But often, I remember her say, like it was yesterday, "Let's hold this or that loosely." She used that phrase often—regarding plans, possessions, even people. "Our hold on these things should be loose."

Now, years later and in a long season of "letting go," Carol's intelligent words of old are new to me, over and over, and some of the wisest words I've ever heard. Carol herself has become a pro at letting go ... and from afar, we continue to lift each other up in prayer.

Living On a Prayer—September 23, 2011

Everyone and their dog (literally) was at the dike today. Mike and I have been riding our bikes at the dikes a lot lately to avoid traffic and to enjoy the amazing scenery. The Golden Ears Mountains of Maple Ridge were stunning as usual and Mount Baker in all its snowy splendour was so close we could almost touch it even though it's all the way (south across the border) in the USA.

It's been raining on and off for the last few days. I keep saying the humidity reminds me of the Amazon. Mike says this is the way it feels in Toronto after a rainfall. The birds were chirping and the crickets were cricketing and the bugs were sticking to our sweat … what a great day!

We rode the dike from the entrance at Laity Street to Harris Road in Pitt Meadows. We always have to touch the gate at Harris Road or Mike says you can't say you have been all the way. Round trip from our house and back is about 19K. We took a little break at the gate and made fun of each other's sweaty bug collection.

Mike suggested we ride on the other side back. We have only taken that path once and it was so bumpy, I'm sure I had a concussion by the end of it … maybe just whip lash, but it wasn't very enjoyable, so I told Mike no. Then I thought, whatever Mike wants, Mike should get. So I said, "Your wish is my command."

His one eyebrow raised and with a frisky look on his face, he said, "In that case, I will save my wish for later." So, we rode back the way we came.

As we started out, Mike said we were halfway there, which reminded me of the song, "Living on a Prayer."

"Who sings that, again?" I asked Mike.

"Bon Jovi."

As we pedalled, he thought about his wish for tonight (I could tell by the look on his face), and I thought about the goodness of God and how He hears our prayers and always answers. Sometimes His answer is "no"; sometimes it is "yes"; and sometimes it's "not now."

With all the ALS discoveries and breakthroughs in the news lately, we are growing more and more excited. We are a little nervous as well ... what if the cure isn't discovered soon enough? So, like the song says, we are living on a prayer and believe that God's timing is always perfect ... whatever happens!

While Elanna and I were chatting earlier today, she quoted Philippians 4:6-7, "Do not be anxious about anything, but in everything, by prayer and petition, with thanksgiving, present your requests to God. And the peace of God, which transcends all understanding, will guard your hearts and your minds in Christ Jesus."

Half Handicapped—September 24, 2011—by Mike Sands

Question: What's the difference between a Scottish guy and a water fountain? Answer: You can get a drink out of a water fountain.

That's a racist joke, but I'm half Scottish, so society allows me to say it without me being considered a racist. An episode of *The Jeffersons* had George Jefferson going to court to pay a speeding ticket. When George entered the courtroom, he noticed a lot of black defendants there. He said in a loud voice, "There's enough niggers in here to make a Tarzan movie." Not only did George use the "n" word, he used it on television. Not only would any non-black person be considered a racist if they said that word, the CRTC, the FCC, FBI, and a whole bunch of other Alphagetti Agencies would revoke the television station's licence immediately.

I've had ALS for just over a year now. They tell me the illness starts out slowly with muscle weakness, slurred speech, and muscle atrophy, all of which I have experienced. I also have a stiff gait, and my right hand is down to about 20 percent usage.

It's kind of funny watching people's reaction to you when you're progressing toward full incapacitation. One time at the bank, the teller said to me, "Oh, your hand looks sore." Another time I accidentally staggered into a guy's car when he was at a stop sign. He rolled the window down and stated, "What are you, drunk or something? You just bumped into my car." A more civilized response would have been, "Are you okay?"

This is why I consider myself "Half-handicapped," because at this stage of the illness it is hard to distinguish whether I'm just not well (i.e. injured or intoxicated) or whether I am handicapped.

They tell me after the second year of the illness, most patients are wheelchair bound. That means, if it goes according to their schedule, I should be in a wheelchair next summer.

Before I go, I have one more joke for you. How many handicapped people does it take to screw in a lightbulb? I'll tell you the punch line next summer.

Separation Anxiety—September 26, 2011

Our two-year-old dog Molly, a robust (some would say "fat"), medium-sized, brindle-coloured, mixed breed, was acting a little strangely a couple of weeks ago. She seemed a little sad … she just wasn't herself. I found her lying in the front yard, holding Madison's shoe in her paw, the way a small child sleeping on her tummy would hold her favourite teddy bear. I told Mike about it and he said that Molly was probably chewing on Madison's shoe. Madison and I had both left a pair of running shoes on the front porch to dry out after a day of river rafting with Madison's hockey team. Molly thinks that shoes left outside are free game. She leaves the ones inside alone, but has destroyed most of those left outside.

I took another look to make sure Molly wasn't eating Madison's shoe. I saw her holding it, rubbing her head against it, sticking her nose in it, and laying her cheek on it … she definitely wasn't chewing it. I'm no expert, but I'm pretty sure Molly was experiencing separation anxiety. Madison had just gone back to school and Molly was having some difficulty adjusting to Madison's new schedule.

I think I have been experiencing separation anxiety as well. I'm not carrying around Mike's shoe, but I do find I become anxious when I'm apart from him.

Eight months ago, Mike was working a lot, so he wasn't home very much and when he did come home, it wasn't for long. Apart from doing his laundry, I didn't have to worry about him. He ate at work and mostly fended for himself. Now, Mike is home full time and dealing with some limitations. With my part-time job and a few other commitments, I have to go out without Mike almost every day. I find I worry a little after an hour and a half or two hours go by. What if he needs me to fix him a snack, or help him put on a shirt, or scratch his back, or open a can of spaghetti sauce? What if he loses his footing and slips on the stairs, or trips over the shoe Molly dropped in the middle of the living room floor? Mike says he is fine and that I shouldn't worry, but adjusting to my "half handicapped" husband's new limitations is challenging and sometimes a little stressful.

I am happy to report, Molly is doing much better. She waits patiently for Madison to come home from school, now that she knows Madison will be back soon. I am doing okay as well ... Mike waited patiently for me today to come home so I could open a can of spaghetti sauce. He had the noodles cooked and the beef browned and a big smile on his face. He assured me he didn't mind waiting ... he knew I'd be back soon.

Newsworthy—September 29, 2011

Mike received a phone call the day before yesterday from a reporter from the *Maple Ridge News*. Robert had seen my blog and was interested in meeting us. Mike told him to come on over and after he hung up, he asked me what I thought he might want. I told Mike he probably wants to do a story. Mike was a little confused and said, "I have ALS, but I don't think it's newsworthy."

Robert came over yesterday and he was younger and less serious than I thought he would be for an award-winning journalist. After he introduced himself, he asked if I was George Klassen's daughter. He said he had done a number of articles on my mom and dad and their adventures in Malawi, Africa drilling wells and taking care of orphans. He took his shoes off before I could tell him not to, and had a seat.

Robert became a friend right away. It didn't seem like he was doing a job; it felt like we already knew him and he was just dropping by to say hi.

He said he had read some of our posts and wanted to know what inspired me to start the blog. I told him I wanted friends and family to be able to know how Mike is doing. I told Robert that Mike's family live in Toronto and that maybe a blog would be a good way for them to stay connected to the son and brother they adore. I also said that Mike has such a positive attitude and great sense of humour that if I could inspire or encourage some people by writing about Mike, then that would be well worth it. Robert suggested that perhaps someone recently diagnosed with ALS would benefit from reading my blog as well. I told him I really hoped so.

Robert asked lots of questions. He asked Mike about his work and Mike liked that. Robert wanted to know why Mike became a nurse and asked if Mike felt nursing was a rewarding job and if he enjoyed it. Without any hesitation, Mike said, "YES, absolutely!" and he explained how nursing was a "calling." Robert wanted to know about our travels to Africa with Project Wellness, the charitable organization our family founded. He wanted to know about Mike's biking and inquired about the few accidents he'd read about in my blog. He asked about our children and how we are all handling the situation. We told him we have our moments, of course, but we keep looking up.

Toward the end of our visit, Mike shared how he is surprised that he isn't as sad as he thinks he should be after receiving such horrible news. He said it has to do with the peace of knowing God and the comfort of knowing there is something better to come.

Oswald Chamber writes a passage titled, "The Source of Abundant Joy," on March 7 (the day Mike was diagnosed with ALS) in his *My Utmost for His Highest*, "The underlying foundation of the Christian faith is the undeserved, limitless miracle of the love of God that was exhibited on the Cross of Calvary; a love that is not earned and never can be ... And the experiences of life, whether they are everyday events or terrifying ones, are powerless to 'separate us from the love of God.'"

You're The Best, Man—October 1, 2011

Mike was honoured when our son Nathan asked him to be his best man. "Best man" pretty much sums it up. Best is best. There is good, then better, then best.

Here are a few reasons why his son and two daughters might think he is the best. First of all, he is the greatest trick-or-treater on the planet. I can still see their little faces watching in awe as Mike shared his secrets to collecting at least twice as much candy as the other kids. They were also amazed how he could throw the insides of the pumpkin in a pan and put it in the oven and after a half hour or so, pull out a beautiful pie. He got away with the trick a couple of times before they clued in that Mike quickly made the switch when he sent them off to play ... Mike still denies it.

Mike played with his children at the park, and never let the ice cream guy go by without buying three cool treats or more depending on how many friends were in tow. Sometimes he set up his own ice cream stand and, with the help of our children, he would sell ice cream cones to the neighbour kids for one cent a cone ... his motto was "we will not be undersold." It wasn't unusual to have ten to twenty kids lined up to place their order at our kitchen window. Jared, the boy from across the street would come with a dime to pick up dessert for his whole family.

Mike was never too busy to tell a story, solve a problem, or patch a wound. Road hockey, a little baseball and kicking the soccer ball around was part of their regular routine. Mike helped them with their homework and skipped them (and friends) out of school to see their favourite movies.

Even with Mike's hectic work schedule, he managed to make most of their games, track and cross country meets, public speaking competitions, plays, and school band concerts.

Roller coasters and roller blades, water slides and water fights … Mike was like a big friend. Mike is still a friend, just not as big now that they are almost all grown up.

Even though Mike never followed the Dr. Spock principles of child rearing, his son and daughters think his methods were best. And to prove it, this past August, proud as punch, Mike stood beside his boy and was the best "best man" a son could have.

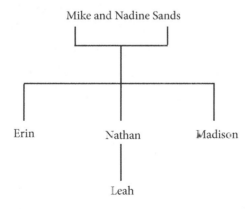

"Start children off on the way they should go,
and even when they are old they will not turn from it."
Proverbs 22:6

Half Nelson—October 3, 2011

Our bus driver Bruce was a nice enough guy, but he drove really slowly, which was annoying and he kept pumping the brakes going downhill, which made me feel nauseated. Mike pointed out that Bruce looked like *Bowling for Columbine*'s Michael Moore and the coach pointed out that he talked way too much and Leighton pointed out the window and said, "Hey look, we are actually passing someone." I looked out and saw the two cyclists he was referring to, pedalling up the hill beside us. Leighton is one of the hockey dads and the equipment manager who provides a little comic relief.

Well, it's hockey season and we are on the road again. We left for the 600 km trip to Nelson on Friday at 5:00 a.m. After three wins, zero losses, and a few bumps and bruises (no major injuries), we headed back Sunday morning.

It's Madison's last year with the Fraser Valley Phantoms, a major midget hockey team that plays in the BC female hockey league. Mike was glad he could join us and plans to come on all the road trips this year; I already go on all the road trips because I'm the team trainer/safety person. In past seasons, Mike didn't make many hockey trips (Nathan's or Madison's), because he had to work.

Mike was happy when he heard our first trip was to Nelson, because he could make a bunch of "half Nelson" jokes. He told my parents we would give them a call from "half Nelson." He suggested a few times that we should stop for lunch at "half Nelson" and so on.

Mike is kind of famous around our house for "the half nelson"—a wrestling term for an arm twist behind the back. He is also famous for "the Vulcan"—the tight squeeze of his hand on the collarbone; the "backache"—knuckle between the shoulder blades; the "toe crack"—just like it sounds; and "the Terry"—an ear pull. Mike adopted the Terry one day when he saw a mother pulling her child by the ear saying, "Terry, it's your birthday, get back to the party."

Mike would often put one of the kids or me in one of the above vice grips and tell us to say, "Uncle Mike's the greatest." He wouldn't let go until those words were spoken. The kids would resist and take the torture for a while, not wanting to give their dad the satisfaction of hearing "Uncle Mike's the greatest." I would simply say, "I don't have an Uncle Mike, but sure, I'll say it." And I would oblige.

The beautiful town of Nelson is located in the Kootenays of British Columbia. The last time we were there was last March, the weekend before Mike was diagnosed. We were a little anxious about the appointment, but nevertheless we had a great time that weekend, watching the last league hockey games of the season and socializing at Finley's Pub with the other parents and coaches. We also took a few walks in the snow and prayed about the neurologist visit.

After Mike was diagnosed, we always said that "Mike has been *diagnosed* with ALS." It's only recently, we say "he *has* ALS." But that shouldn't fool anyone. Mike still believes that he could have been misdiagnosed, because anything is possible. He is even more convinced that he could be miraculously healed or that a cure could come at any time ... because anything is possible with God.

In a little convenience store in Half Nelson—some small town about half way there—I bought a rock with the words, "All things are possible with God."

One and a Half Handicapped—October 6, 2011

It was our niece Heather's birthday on Monday. Heather is Pat and Gary's daughter. She lives in Langley with her hubby Frank and their beautiful five-year-old daughter Kaelyn who started kindergarten this fall. Heather had an appointment in White Rock and not only was it her birthday, but the forecast called for rain and because Heather has Cerebral Palsy, she was going to have to take her wheelchair on a connect-the-dots bus trip to her appointment, so we offered to take her. We gave ourselves about forty-five minutes to get there, but it only took fifteen. It would have taken Heather about an hour and a half by busses.

Most of the parking in front of the building was handicapped parking. Mike told me to park in one of the handicapped spots. He and Heather both agreed that even though I don't have a permit to park in a handicapped spot, it was more than okay because, after all, they were "one and a half handicapped." Instead, I dropped them off and parked somewhere else. I had a flashback of the Seinfeld episode where George parks in a handicap spot and when he, Elaine, Kramer, and Jerry return to the car, it's been destroyed by a mob of angry people. I'm glad I parked somewhere else, because when we came out after the appointment, all the handicapped spots were taken and it was easy for me to go get the car and come back for my one and a half handicapped passengers.

Mike is doing well adjusting to his half handicap … but here is a question: Is it more difficult for a person to become handicapped later on in life, or to be born that way and never know the difference?

We dropped Heather off with time for her to go pick Kaelyn up from school. Later, Mike and I went back to Langley with Nathan and Leah to take Heather, Frank, and Kaelyn out for birthday dinner. Frank is a bike expert … sales, service etc. He took Mike's bike last week to make a few adjustments. When we met them for dinner, Frank had Mike's bike ready for him. He's switched the brakes, so now the back brake is on the left handlebar—Mike's strong side. He also put on new tires, tuned it up, and presented Mike with a brand new helmet (we are pretty sure the helmet is a contribution from Pat).

Today, while Mike and I were out running a few errands, I paid extra attention to how people responded to Mike's half handicap. A woman at the doctor's office seemed a little annoyed when she had to move over coming up the stairs for Mike who needed the left handrail while going down the stairs. Someone at the drug store seemed a little impatient because we were walking slowly and they obviously had to get somewhere fast. At the grocery store, Mike likes to push the buggy because it helps him with his balance, but others who had better things to do seemed a little antsy when Mike couldn't steer his buggy out of their way fast enough. Mike thinks he should wear a hat that says, "I have ALS," so people will perhaps be more sympathetic.

In Heather's case, it's a little more obvious, but I'm guessing she has always experienced similar responses.

As I observed my one and a half handicapped passengers, humbled, I realized that I need to be more patient with others less capable than me and more grateful for my capabilities.

Happy Giving—October 10, 2011

Today, while driving home from Point Grey after dropping Erin off at her place, I contemplated the events of this Thanksgiving weekend.

It was raining and by the way people were driving, you would think it never rains. We live in Vancouver ... it rains more than it doesn't. I explained to Mike and Madison a few times, that I could understand people wanting to slow down in the rain, but "PLEASE get out of the fast lane!" In between my impatient outbursts, I was giving thanks ... really.

We had a delicious salmon dinner yesterday instead of the traditional turkey spread. My parents had us all over and served the fish my dad caught while they were in Port Hardy last month. We were all there except Madison, who got a call last minute from a friend to play hockey. Mike left early to watch some of the game and when my dad found out that Mike had left for the game, he quickly gobbled the last couple of bites on his plate and flew out the door with Nathan to catch the last period. They all came back, including Madison, just in time for warm apple pie and ice cream.

Last year, I was in the Dominican Republic on Thanksgiving. I was missing my family, but was experiencing a little more gratitude than usual. I was there for two weeks with a group of people in the construction business and in the business of giving and helping, including my cousin Brian. My parents decided I should go. Through Project Wellness, they had already donated the funds for two homes in a village and were sponsoring two more homes in a new village. So, I was sent to help with the construction of these houses and to visit the recipients of the houses Project Wellness has provided. We were putting tin roofs on brick houses.

I had been on a few Project Wellness mission trips before—to Brazil, Nigeria, and Malawi (Mike and the kids have all been to Malawi as well). But none were like this one. The others were more geared toward helping out in churches, visiting orphans, hospital visitation, education, delivering medication, soccer balls, and jerseys, etc. This trip was about physical work ... blood, sweat, and tears. Okay, not so much blood and tears, but a lot of sweat ... and a few tears.

Our young and fearless leader Josh had a birthday while we were there. I didn't know Josh before the trip, but only a few days in, I felt like I had known him for a long time; he quickly became a friend ... with everyone in the group. While speaking with him at dinner the night before his birthday, I heard that quiet voice inside me say, "Give him your book." I continued my conversation with Josh while I had a little talk with the Spirit inside me.

The book He was referring to was my favourite copy of *My Utmost for His Highest* by Oswald Chambers ... a dear possession. My dad gave me my first copy years ago. It stayed in a drawer for a long time before I took it out and discovered the riches inside. It is now crammed in between other books in my bookcase. The copy I took with me to the Dominican, that I felt the Lord was now asking me to give away, was a revised edition I had been reading for years. It was well worn, like a favourite pair of sweat pants you put on when you want to get comfortable. It was marked with pen, pencil, highlighter, even eyeliner—in all the right places. Pages were torn, folded, and falling out. Some would consider it trash; it was treasure to me.

Giving my book to Josh was difficult and a little embarrassing; he probably thought it was weird. It was easier for me to give two weeks of my time, effort, and sweat and tears in the construction of those homes than it was to give my tattered and torn, soft-covered book away (retail value, $4.99).

Just before I presented it to the birthday boy, I opened it up to take my last look inside, and this is what Oswald said: "Wherever God sends us, He will guard our lives. Our personal property and possessions are to be a matter of indifference to us, and our hold on these things should be very loose."

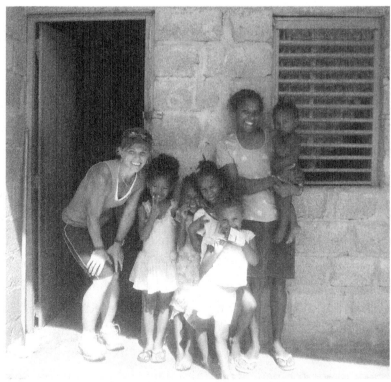

Nadine with happy home recipients
in the Dominican Republic

~ ~ ~ ~ ~ ~

Our hold on all things should be loose, indeed. Like Job said, "Naked I came from my mother's womb, and naked I will depart. The Lord gave and the Lord has taken away; may the name of the Lord be praised," (Job 1:21).

One might question if the Lord actually "takes away." Would a loving God take all of those things away from Job, a man the Lord described as blameless and upright, a man who feared God and shunned evil?

The thing is Job had everything and then he had nothing. He was stripped of beloved people and all of his possessions, and laid bare before a few friends and God. But tested and tried, Job's true colours shone through. Job 1:22 says, "In all this, Job did not sin by charging God with wrongdoing."

God is sovereign. Ultimately, He is in control. He decides what comes and goes in our lives and when and why. We may not understand, but that's what faith is for. We have a pea in our heads compared to the knowledge and wisdom of God ... Our tiny brains can't comprehend the mind of Him, but that's what faith is for.

My friend Carol's faith and wise instruction to "hold things loosely" have been tested over and over again in her own life. Physically yes, but so much more painful than the agony she lives in with a degenerative tendon disorder in her feet and hands, she has had to let go of her oldest son. Not to college away from home or a career in another country or marriage and a family of his own, but to a life on the streets, to the many fails at rehab, to crime and jail-time, and all that a life of addiction entails.

She has had to let go a million times. It's the ultimate test of her lesson to "hold all things loosely." She "holds him loosely," her own son and she clings to the only One who's got it all under control.

And may the name of the Lord be praised!

Chapter 3
Slippery Slope

The first time I went to GF Strong Rehabilitation Hospital was in 1993 to visit my uncle Eugene. He spent a few months there after falling down the stairs in his home and damaging his spinal cord. He was a strong, healthy man on June 17 and on June 18, a quadriplegic.

We all lose our footing from time to time, but this slip of the foot brought devastation; instant paralysis ... and it was just an accident!

Mike's paralysis, though not an accident but an incurable disease, is gradual. His letting go of everything comes in stages; my uncle's was immediate.

These men, I'm sure would say, be thankful for today ... you never know what tomorrow may bring.

Dream Team—October 11, 2011

Mike had an appointment last week with the ALS Team at GF Strong in Vancouver. Instead of seeing the neurologist this time, he saw the occupational therapist, speech therapist, dietician, the ALS nurse, social worker, and the gadget lady (another occupational therapist specializing in helping ALS patients find ways of maintaining independence). Mike was excited to purchase a knife from the gadget lady. It's a long, sharp knife you hold like a saw. The first time he used it, he said, "It works really well, and I only cut myself three times."

Elanna came with us to the appointment. She has come to all three appointments at GF Strong since Mike was diagnosed. She provides emotional support, she asks questions we forget to ask, and she always brings a bag of snacks. We call ourselves the "Dream Team" ... we are dreaming that we will show up and the doctor will say something like, "Sorry for the inconvenience, Mr. Sands, but we have made a mistake and you don't have ALS after all. You are free to go."

We can dream, right?

It was a three-and-a-half-hour appointment this time. The ALS Team asked every question in the book.

"How is your swallowing?

"How are you managing in the shower?

"How is your breathing?

"How are you managing going up and down the stairs?

"What is the layout of your house?

"Are you eating softer foods?

"Are you choking, are you sleeping, are you coughing, are you able to dress yourself, can you brush your teeth, can you balance on one leg, are you still able to leap tall buildings in a single bound?"

It was emotionally draining, because answering all the questions was a reminder of all the changes in our lives caused by the illness and all the changes yet to come. Even though we were exhausted, Mike and Elanna still had enough energy when we left to act out a scene from a horror movie with Mike's new knife.

The changes can sometimes be overwhelming, but the things that stay the same bring comfort and joy. Mike is still the same on the inside and that will never change.

Last night I listened to Mike give Madison a lesson on the Treaty of Versailles with all the knowledge and passion he has for history, and although he speaks more slowly and words are slurred, he still speaks with the eloquence and conviction he's always had.

This morning, while at the fruit and vegetable market, Mike made the same old jokes about "squeezing my melons" and "holding my melons" and "maybe looking for larger melons" and so forth.

Later, Mike went for a bike ride and when he returned, like a kid, he was happy to show off the dirt that covered him from head to toe. He had gone 13K in the rain and was wearing that mud like a badge or a ribbon or a medal or something. What an accomplishment!

"Courage is the power to let go of the familiar."
Raymond Lindquist

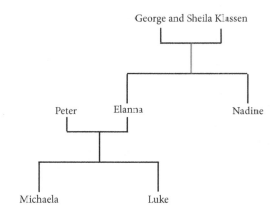

Larger Melons—October 12, 2011

I didn't sleep well last night, plus I gave it all I had in my spin class this morning, even though I have a cold, so today after lunch I had to lie down for a few minutes.

Just as I put my head on the pile of unfolded laundry on the couch, I heard Mike say, "Well, I'm ready for a bike ride now."

What? I am way too tired, I thought, plus it was way too cold and it looked like it could rain. Do I tell him I don't want to go? Do I tell him I can't go? Do I pretend I've been bit by a venomous spider and I can't move my body? But I didn't want to let Mike down, so I dragged myself off the couch and put on a second pair of socks, a heavy sweater, and a long jacket. I guess I didn't look that enthusiastic because when we left Mike said, "I don't think you really want to go."

Mike continues to inspire me every day. He never complains, he never whines, it's never "woe is me." I, however whined for the first ten minutes of our bike ride, but eventually I warmed up and decided to enjoy every minute with my beloved. And just like he said, I didn't need the long jacket. We talked and joked and every five minutes we had to stop so I could put on or take off another layer of clothing.

During our quiet times, I just thought about stuff. I thought about Mike and my larger melon discussion at the market the other day and how he always makes me laugh. I thought about how I need to get a case for Mike's new knife, because I threw the knife in my bag when we went out for lunch today and when the server showed up with Mike's steak sandwich I reached in to get the knife and almost lost a finger. I thought about all the new movies that showed up in a package today from Pat … I was particularly excited about the *Get Smart Season 2* DVD. I thought how Mike is in such good shape even though he has a terminal illness and how that—along with his positive attitude and strong faith—will contribute to his quality of life and will most definitely extend his life as well. I thought about many things and as we pulled up in the driveway, I thought how I wouldn't have wanted to miss that bike ride with Mike for anything!

My "R" Rated Blog—October 17, 2011—by Mike Sands

The reason this blog is "R" rated is because some of the pictures are very graphic and may be disturbing to some readers.

I went for a bike ride on the dike a couple of days ago and had an accident. A dog walked in front of my bike and I went for a spill. When I hit the dog, he hardly moved because I wasn't going very fast. Unfortunately for me, my co-ordination and reflexes are not as quick as they were before ALS. I have difficulty catching myself, so my knees and face took the brunt of the fall. My sister had just bought me an expensive helmet the week before, after she heard of my previous accident. I didn't have my new helmet on, because I thought I wouldn't need it for the dike where there are no cars. After falling, I had to pedal about seven miles back home. All I could think of was how much my sister was going to give me heck for not wearing my helmet.

After I showered off the blood, I noticed my nose was broken. My doctor told me to meet him at the hospital. He said he would stuff cocaine up my nose and set it (cocaine is the drug of choice for nasal work, as it dulls the pain and is a vasodilator).

While in the emergency room at the hospital with Nadine and

Elanna, we had a good laugh over the day's events. I decided I would write a story for Nadine's blog. We went over different titles for the blog and these are a few we came up with: Look Away, I'm Hideous Part 2; Scarface 2; Nose to the Grindstone; and Dog Day Afternoon.

I got back on my bike the next day. I must admit though, these past biking accidents have made me more tentative, but biking is my only means of exercise now, because I can't run or lift weights anymore ... "So look out fear, I'm passing on the left!"

To my sister Pat—I will wear my helmet all the time, even on the dike.

Mine is Only Rated "PG"—October 18, 2011

I came home on Thursday after my hair appointment excited to tell Mike that when I went to pay for my haircut, the lady at the till told me it had already been taken care of. I knew right away that it was either my mom or my sister who'd gone ahead of me and paid. It was such a nice surprise, unlike the surprise I got when I went upstairs to tell Mike about it.

I heard the shower running and figured Mike had just gotten back from his bike ride. I went into the bathroom and right away sensed something was wrong. I asked Mike from my side of the curtain if everything was okay and he said nothing. I looked at his clothes lying on the floor and saw blood. My heart sank.

I go bike riding with Mike almost every day and the day I go to the salon instead, he has another accident. Mike and I have an agreement ... or so I thought. When I don't go riding with

Chapter 3

him, he goes to the dirt track at the high school just down the road at Merkley Park. I feel comfortable with that arrangement. He doesn't have to cross any busy roads, there are no hills, there is no traffic, etc. I thought I convinced him that the dike and other bike trips are best taken together. But like a rebellious child, Mike disobeyed and went to the dike by himself.

He explained that a dog walked across his path and even though he slowed down, he was unable to steer around the dog and, because of his loss of range of motion and strength in his arms, he was unable to catch himself before he hit the ground with his face. So, needless to say, it was another "Look Away, I'm Hideous" moment all over again. A little worse though, Mike broke his nose ... the dog was fine. I convinced Mike to see the doctor and his nose was taken care of.

All Mike could think about was the great pictures he got and the blog he was going to write. All I could think about was his family in Toronto and how upset they were going to be when they read about the incident. I insisted he keep the accident under wraps, but nothing can keep Mike from telling a good story ... especially one that involves blood. I pleaded with him to leave it alone, but he had his mind made up.

When I woke up this morning, I lay in bed and prayed for Mike's family. I prayed that the Lord would comfort them and help them not to worry about their little brother too much.

When I got up, this is the message I read from Mike's sister Aileen: "Mike's R Rated blog post made me cry, but I think it is selfish of me to think about my feelings when I see my brother handling himself so strongly and never giving up or giving in. It's sad for us to see him suffer anything, but there is such a message in his story that caused me to really think

43

deeply about what it means to him to continue the biking in spite of the dangers. He doesn't want to give his whole being to ALS and continuing this activity shows how he is continuing with his life as he always has—with strength, endurance, and a whole lot of faith."

Aileen's message to Mike: "Hey Mike, I just want you to know that every day you amaze me with your strength of person and humour at life and its hurdles. You have taught me so much; inspiration, yes, but more about growing stronger in spirit in the face of barriers. It is again you heading face on (literally) to your limitations and not letting them rob you of your pleasures. I love that you can laugh at this; the pictures are priceless, and they show who you are and NOBODY would change that in you. I just hate that you got hurt."

"An invincible determination can accomplish anything and in that, lies the great distinction between great men and little men."
Thomas Fuller

In Sickness and in Health—October 20, 2011

Today, while I stretched Mike out and gave him a massage, I watched the show, *Say Yes to the Dress*. It really struck me when the commentator said, "Choosing the right dress, isn't always easy." My first thought was, How about choosing the right partner?

The very excited and perhaps slightly naïve bride lists the features she is looking for in a dress: traditional, strapless, sweetheart neckline, with beading, etc. I watched and wondered if she made a list of the qualities she is looking for in a husband as well: honest, hardworking, sensitive, romantic ... And does she know that even if "Mr. Right" meets all the requirements on her list, there is no guarantee that the marriage is going to always go well? Any married person would agree that the only guarantee in a marriage is that there will be rough patches.

Someone recently said to me that Mike and I are lucky to have such a good marriage. Lucky? What? It has nothing to do with luck! It does have a lot to do with God's grace and answered prayer, though. It also has a lot to do with hard work, sacrifice, commitment, and a bunch of other stuff.

I didn't have a list of features I wanted in a wedding dress, because I didn't wear a wedding dress when I got married. I wore pink pants and a white blouse when we said our vows in Los Angeles where Mike and I eloped. I didn't have a list of qualities I wanted in a husband either, because I was in love and that was good enough ... I was an excited, naïve bride as well.

I got married at nineteen, had a baby at twenty, and one day woke up and wondered what had happened. At one time, I had three children under the age of six, I was running a business, and teaching thirteen fitness classes a week ... I was a little tired to say the least. Doing another load of laundry wasn't that difficult, but keeping the home fires burning was. And when Mike went to school and worked evenings, my needs went out the window. To be totally honest, the grass did look greener on the other side sometimes.

As Mike and I walked and talked and pondered life together a few days before Mike was diagnosed with ALS, he said, "They say the grass is always greener on the other side .... Well, I guess I'm on the other side then." We have dodged some bullets and have said a lot of prayers and are one of the "lucky" couples that have made it this far.

Mike and I haven't been on a date for a while and I can't remember the last candlelit dinner, but today I stretched out his hamstrings and he said it really helped—he was able to put his socks on. Now that's wedded bliss!

The Georges and Sheilas of Our Lives—October 22, 2011

I received a phone message from my mom the other day. The message started with her singing one of her favourite songs by Stevie Wonder: "I just called to say I love you, I just called to say I care, I just called to say I love you … and I mean it from the bottom of my heart." She went on to say, "If you need anything, just let me know." And she signed off with her signature goodbye; "Chow" (really spelled "ciao").

My mom's name is Sheila and Mike's mum's name is Sheila as well; (the "mom" versus "mum" isn't a typo; my mom is "Mom" and Mike's is "Mum"). Our moms having the same name might not be that unusual, but here's what's unusual—our dads have the same name as well—George.

Having parents with the same names made it easy for us to name our children: Erin Sheila, Nathaniel George, and Madison Sheila. In private, Mike tells his parents we named the kids after them and privately he tells my parents we named the kids after them.

Anyway, hearing my Sheila sing made me smile. Hearing her voice and her reminder, "If you need anything, I am here for you," brings so much comfort. Hearing Mike's Sheila's voice makes me smile too. She has a lovely Scottish accent that makes me want to listen … even to stories I have heard many times. I can sit and listen to her and her sister Aileen reminisce for hours, recalling childhood memories growing up with their big brothers in Scotland and then immigrating to Canada in 1948.

When I call my parents' house and my George picks up, it's "HI DEE, how are you, Dee?" He has called me "Dee" (or "Dee Dee") all my life. He doesn't want to chat like my mom does, but he takes the time to make me feel like he really cares. As soon as he hears I am well, he says, "Okay, here is your mom. Let me know if you need anything." I was told that when my mom was pregnant with my sister, my dad really wanted a boy. After having a baby girl and falling head over heels for her, he wanted another girl when my mom was pregnant with me. I have always felt incredibly loved.

Mike's George doesn't want to talk long either, he simply wants to hear Mike's voice … to know that Mike is okay and that he and his family are doing well. He is tough on the outside, but on the inside, he is soft. He doesn't say a lot, but you know he is there and you know he cares.

Our Sheilas still feed us and clothe us and slip us cash. Our Georges won't let us pay for anything and they all hate to see us suffer in any way.

The Georges and Sheilas of our lives support us, care for us, love us, encourage us, and treat us like gold. We feel blessed beyond measure!

Telling our parents about Mike's diagnosis was harder than hearing it ourselves. We knew it would devastate them and that it did. But their strength inspires us and they continue to muster up the courage to walk with us through the toughest times of our lives. We love them and thank God for them every day!

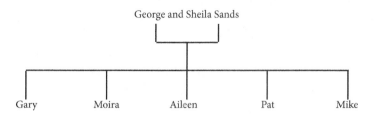

George and Sheila Sands

Gary   Moira   Aileen   Pat   Mike

Mike's Glass is Half Full—October 25, 2011

Today, Mike said to me that there was a positive side to taking so many pills—he gets the recommended eight glasses of water a day. The guy always looks on the bright side.

When the big "horse pill" goes down sideways and he gags it back up, he says he's fine and tries again. He never complains.

Mike's glass is always half full. He is a positive person. When he was diagnosed with ALS, he remained pretty hopeful that he had been misdiagnosed. When the doctor recommended that he stop working and go on long-term disability, he said he could use some time off. When his right hand continued to weaken, he said, "It's a good thing I'm left-handed." When he was unable to run anymore, he was glad he could go for walks. When he gave up going for walks, he was thankful he could still ride his bike. When he fell off his bike and landed on his face (again) and broke his nose, he said that the accident taught him to be more careful next time.

I was attracted to Mike's positive attitude right away, and it's a quality that has blessed me throughout our twenty-three years of marriage. Time and time again, Mike has helped me to put things in perspective and to keep my chin up.

On March 10, only three days after Mike was first diagnosed, I couldn't sleep, so I sat in bed and read. Mike woke up and asked if he could pray for me. He thanked God for choosing me for him, and asked the Lord to make my burdens light (a prayer he continues to pray for me every day). He went on to say that he was thankful for everything, even the things he doesn't want, like ALS. He prayed that he would learn what he is supposed to learn from the very humbling experience of being diagnosed with this illness. He said that this "humbling experience" would cause him to rely more on God.

> *"Never try to live your life with God in any other way than His way. And His way means absolute devotion to Him. Showing no concern for the uncertainties that lie ahead is the secret of walking with Him."*
> **Oswald Chambers**

Just Some Thoughts—October 27, 2011

I have been mad about something for a while now. I don't get mad that easily, but when I do, I find that everything annoys me. Things that don't normally bother me, all of a sudden drive me crazy.

This morning, as I was stewing in my anger and growing more and more agitated, I was very tempted to start thinking about how mad I should be about Mike's illness. I was very close to allowing myself to think about how maddening it is and how furious I could be! I knew if I let myself get mad about the ALS, I would go to a place it would be hard to come back from.

While standing on the edge of a very slippery slope, I was reminded of Philippians 4:8, which says, "Finally, brothers and sisters, whatever is true, whatever is noble, whatever is right, whatever is pure, whatever is lovely, whatever is admirable—if anything is excellent or praiseworthy—think about such things."

I had to redirect my thoughts. I had to loosen my grip on this life and its strife, and grab hold of God and think about things that are excellent and praiseworthy.

While writing this blog post on my laptop in my living room, I looked out the window and saw Nathan and Mike walking home from the park pushing Leah in her stroller. When they came in, Mike proceeded to take chestnuts out of his jacket pocket ... one by one. It took him some time to take all twenty-two chestnuts out of his pockets and place them on the dining room table.

I asked him how the park was and he said they didn't stay at the park for long, they went to the chestnut tree (a tree we visited many times with our children when they were small ... just a little way down the street from the park). I could see that Mike had a lovely time with his son and granddaughter, and it made me happy.

As I continued to type on my laptop, Mike asked, "What are you writing there?"

I said, "Just some thoughts."

He said, "Do they bring you joy?"

I replied with a very definite, "YES!"

~ ~ ~ ~ ~ ~ ~

I was mad on that particular day because Nathan's marriage, which had just started, had ended. The beautiful family he and his wife worked hard to create crashed. Nathan was devastated and so were the rest of us … and I was mad!

Mike's illness was fairly new and I couldn't keep up with the letting go and now I had to let go of a daughter too? I brought her in and then I had to let her out. There was just so much "letting go" and I didn't anticipate this "letting go" and I was mad and really sad at the same time.

Life is full of maddening situations. My uncle lost his footing on a stair one day and in a heartbeat his life was turned upside down; no more working or walking or playing golf with his brother and their buddies; no wrestling with his grandsons and no more camping trips with his wife—there's nothing much more maddening than that!

Seven years to the day of my Uncle Eugene's fall, he returned to hospital. He died from complications due to his condition on June 24, 2000.

I remember my Auntie Vicki sharing with a group of us girls (cousins and aunts), shortly after my uncle's death, that on that particular day she was feeling mad.

I knew she had a legitimate reason to feel mad, but I didn't know what to say … I couldn't relate, but now I can.

Regarding my daughter-in-law, she'll always have a place in my heart!

Chapter 4
Sorrow and Joy

I was introduced to these two early in our ALS journey, long before I blogged about them. The partnership of sorrow and joy is definitely an interesting phenomenon. While I had experienced some sorrow in my life and I had experienced much joy in my life, I had never experienced the two as one before ... at least not like this. Sorrow and joy; the two linked arms and became one, like in a marriage.

It's something not easily described. "Bittersweet" might come close. I eventually blog about it and say they "commingle" in my life and I try to describe the harmonious blend of the polar opposites.

For instance, an ALS death sentence brings so much sorrow, but the new perspective on life brings a lot of joy. And the two coexist in your life. It's like when Mike had to stop working due to the symptoms of ALS, but then we had all this glorious time together.

I'll never forget the first time Carol called me to tell me her son was in jail. I was like, "Really, that's great!" Odd response you would think, but she was just so happy to know where he was; to know he was still alive ... that's sorrow and joy!

Adam and Eve Got Nothin' On Me—October 31, 2011—by Mike Sands

They say Adam and Eve had the perfect marriage. He didn't have to hear about all the guys she could have married and she didn't have to hear about how good a cook his mother was.

Comedian Rodney Dangerfield's marriage was far from ideal, as he was married to an unfaithful, untrusting woman who, in Dangerfield's cliché quote, gave him "no respect." One day, Dangerfield came home and caught his wife in the arms of another man. He shouted to her, "What do you think you're doing?" She turned to her lover and said, "See, I told you he was stupid." Another time Dangerfield said, "I met my wife at the front door one day; she was wearing only a sheer negligée. Unfortunately, she was just coming home."

Dangerfield's wife was not only unfaithful, she also didn't trust him. One day Dangerfield came home with a red smudge on his forehead. His wife shouted at him, "Lipstick!" Dangerfield stated, "No, I was in a terrible accident and I smashed my forehead into the steering wheel."

She said, "Lucky for you!"

In the 1950s, Hollywood instilled the standards of the perfect marriage with Ozzie and Harriet Nelson, and June and Ward Cleaver. In the 1970s, Hollywood realized that these characters were unrealistic and did a 360 with such role models as Archie and Edith Bunker, and later, Dan and Roseanne Conner.

The perfect marriage doesn't have to follow or avoid any of these marriages. No marriage is going to be perfect as we are all imperfect individuals. We can't expect our mate to line up exactly the way we think in every situation and, therefore, there will be conflicts now and again.

We can look to the Bible in I Corinthians to give us a guide to being a good mate, by replacing the word "love" with "mate." "Mate is patient, mate is kind. It is not self-seeking, not easily angered, it always protects, trusts and hopes."

I look at my marriage where the incursion of my illness has brought to the forefront the marriage adage, "in sickness and in health." With the going getting tough, Nadine, my mate, has got going. My illness has made it difficult for me to do regular activities of daily living that I once enjoyed. I have difficulty putting on my socks and, without asking, Nadine is there to give me a hand. When riding our bikes on the dike, she leads the way in safety. She is there to cut up my meat, give me massages, take me to my doctor's appointments, and the list goes on; all on top of doing her regular activities she's always had, such as work. She has exemplified the definition of a good mate from I Corinthians. It is fitting that with Lou Gehrig's disease I quote Gehrig with his famous last words to his New York Yankee fans and friends: "I'm the luckiest guy in the world."

~ ~ ~ ~ ~ ~ ~

There was a lot of sorrow involved in becoming Mike's caregiver. It was very difficult for me to witness the quick decline of his health and to watch him give up his independence, but it was an honour and joy to help and care for him. I was constantly in awe of how graciously he let go.

My Auntie Vicki says to me, "You and Mike have something very special, as I felt Eugene and I did. He was never bitter and didn't complain. It was as if he had found an inner peace. When he used to call me if he needed his itchy nose scratched, for example, with 'I know I'm a pain in the a**, but could you … ?' Every time he said this, I thought to myself, yah maybe, but you're my pain in the a** and I love you for it. I still miss him!"

Sorrow and joy indeed …

Drop Everything and Pray—November 2, 2011

Today, Mike and I dropped everything and prayed together. Prayer is normally a part of our everyday lives, but being extremely busy over the last couple of weeks, we haven't had a decent prayer time together in a while.

Mike prayed first and he moved me deeply as he spoke slowly and thoughtfully. His words were slurred, but sounded beautiful to me and I am sure, exceptionally beautiful to the Lord. After giving thanks, he prayed for things in the order he usually does: our children and granddaughter, our parents, our siblings, and their families, some friends and extended family members, and the orphans in Africa. Somewhere in there, he prayed for me ... that my "burdens would be light." Lastly, he laid his cares down on God's big lap.

Mike kept yawning (yawning is a symptom of ALS), and at one point apologized to God for yawning so much. I could sense the Lord sitting right beside Mike, receiving with love, all of his prayers ... yawns included.

> *"We look upon prayer simply as a means of getting things for ourselves, but the biblical purpose of prayer is that we may get to know God Himself. Be yourself before God and present Him with your problems—the very things that have brought you to your wits' end. But as long as you think you are self-sufficient, you don't need to ask God for anything."*
> **Oswald Chambers**

Mike didn't pray that much differently than any other day, but today I was moved to tears as I listened. He wasn't necessarily out to get anything for himself from the One who could give him everything. Mike was simply "casting his cares upon the Lord" and being himself in the presence of God.

Oswald goes on to say, "Prayer isn't a matter of changing things externally, but one of working miracles in a person's inner nature."

Happiness Is a Way of Life—November 4, 2011

We have a sign hanging on a wall in our house that says, "Happiness is not a destination, it is a way of life." I was thinking the other day how important it is in our society to live a long life. Perhaps there is more emphasis on living a long life than living a happy life. According to *Merriam-Webster*, the definition of "happiness" is "a state of well-being and contentment."

A while ago, Mike and I read a book called *The Healing Code*, by Alexander Loyd, PhD, ND. One of the exercises in the book is to rate how you feel about a particular situation on a scale of one to ten and then use words to describe the feelings associated to that situation and then pray about those feelings. The idea is to change the way you feel about something stressful to reduce the stress in your life and help your body heal.

When Mike and I first started the exercise, I would ask Mike to use words to describe how he felt about his illness. He used words like anxious, worried, scared, sad, and helpless. Over time, the words he used were a little anxious, a little bit sad, a little bit worried, and a little bit scared. On July 13, I recorded in my journal the only word Mike used to describe how he felt about his illness, and that word was "content." I think it's interesting that even though Mike wouldn't and didn't use the word "happy" to describe how he felt about his illness, he used the word "content," which is a word used in the definition of happiness.

The apostle Paul says in Philippians 4:12-13, "I know what it is to be in need, and I know what it is to have plenty. I have learned the secret of being content in any and every situation.... I can do everything through Him who gives me strength."

Mike wasn't and still isn't surrendering to ALS; he is trying to live the best life he can in spite of it. He has always been a happy person … content in most situations and ALS can't take that away from him.

Erin recently had a picture on her Facebook page with the words, "What ALS Can't Do: It cannot shatter hope. It cannot destroy peace. It cannot corrode faith. It cannot suppress memories. It cannot conquer the spirit. It cannot silence courage. It cannot invade the soul."

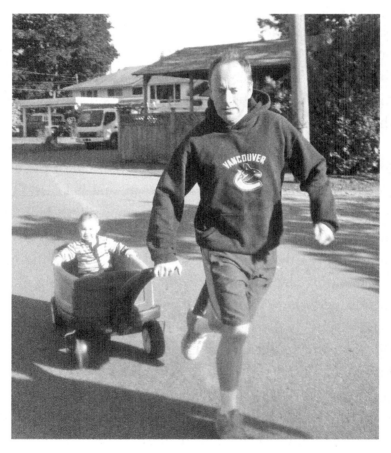

Mike having fun with Leah

This morning when we woke up, I observed Mike as he struggled to get out of bed. Once he finally sat up, he slowly stood up and made his way to the bathroom. I thought how amazing it is that even though Mike's life is changing drastically, in ways that would perhaps fill most of us with fear, he is content … he is happy. It really puts things in perspective for me and I am convicted and humbled once again.

Man of Steel—November 9, 2011

On Monday night, Mike and I went to the Healing Room at the Maple Ridge Community Church. The Healing Room isn't so much about a room; it's more about a group of people who pray. They come together once a week to pray for the needs of anyone who walks through the door. We have been to the Healing Room once before … actually twice, but the first time we went in August, they were closed. So we just prayed together outside on the steps of the church.

Ida, who prayed for us last time, greeted us at the door and asked us to have a seat. While we waited to go into a room where we would receive prayer, Ida chatted with us. Ida asked Mike how he was doing. He said, "About the same."

She said she was hoping to hear he was doing better. He said to her, "Well, the same is better than worse."

She smiled and agreed. She asked him if he was hoping for a miracle.

He said, "Not necessarily; I just want God to be there with me every step of the way."

She again smiled with her very lovely smile and gave a confident look that said, "He is with you and He will never leave you." She looked at me and asked me if I was hoping for a miracle.

I said, "Absolutely!"

We talked for a few more minutes and then were asked to join the prayer team waiting for us in the next room.

Mike and I went in and sat down. I knew three out of the four women on the prayer team. I got up and gave my friend Jennie a big hug, I was so glad to see her. I know Jennie and her husband Brian from the prayer meetings I used to attend at the municipal hall with two other prayer mentors of mine, Eric and Violet.

The room we gathered in was small with subdued lighting. The ladies apologized because the room was so cold. They explained that they were unable to operate the thermostat. I told them it was fine because Mike is a really warm person; I knew Mike would appreciate the cool air.

One of the ladies put a chair in the middle of the room and asked Mike to have a seat. They asked if it was okay for them to lay their hands on him while they prayed. With one of Jennie's hands on my shoulder and all other hands laid on Mike, including mine, they took turns praying, and with passion, compassion, and power, they prayed up a storm. One of the women stood right in front of Mike and took his hands in hers and prayed for his hands. She grabbed hold of his arms and legs, and prayed for his limbs. She placed her hands on his chest and head and prayed for his mind and body. She called him a "man of steel," which I thought was very fitting because Superman is called a "man of steel," and Mike is like Superman to me. At one point Mike became teary. I explained to the ladies that Mike isn't sad. I told them that one of the symptoms of ALS is heightened emotions.

When they were finished praying, one of the women turned to me and said, "You are very strong." She said it again and told me that God knows how strong I am. Then she quoted a verse from the Bible that has been on my mind a lot lately, "When I am weak, He is strong." She told me to remember that when I can't be strong, the Lord will be my strength. Before we left, they broke out into song. They sounded like a chorus of angels as they sang to Mike, "Oh how He loves you, Oh, how He loves you, Oh, how He loves you and me."

When we left, Mike told me that he didn't get choked up because he was upset about the disease; instead, he was moved by the kindness of the women and the presence of God. On the drive home, he told me that he hopes that God heals him just so those nice ladies would be encouraged and for the sake of all the other people that want it for him so badly. He said he didn't know if he wanted it badly enough. He said he didn't feel like it was a life or death situation. He is looking more and more forward to the life beyond this one.

"Valour is stability, not of legs and arms, but of courage and the soul."
Michel de Montaigne

Poof ... You're a New Man—November 12, 2011

Mike was exceptionally slow on Thursday—his movements and his speech. He said he was very jittery and his muscles were really stiff. I could tell he was struggling more than usual. At one point, we were getting ready to go for a bike ride and Mike said he needed to go lie down. I joined him and we read together and I gave him a neck massage.

After a little while, Mike said he was ready to go for a bike ride, but he didn't want to go all the way to the dike today. He told me he would just go down the street to Merkley Park.

Instead of riding my bike with Mike, I walked over with Molly. When Molly and I got to the park, Mike was well into his ride. Molly and I walked across the running track toward the dirt track and I could see Mike in the distance. At first glance, I thought Mike had been healed—he looked like the Mike I've always known. He didn't look like a sick person. He was moving so fast. There were no jitters, no stiffness, no limitations. He looked like he was floating on air and as we got closer I could see a grin from ear to ear.

I threw the ball for Molly in the middle of the grass field and watched Mike ride through the leaves and under the beautiful coloured trees. After about ten laps, he pulled over and joined us. I told him he didn't look like a guy with ALS. He smiled and told me to watch him as he walked around me. He said he felt much better and showed off his smoother gait.

Mike told me he thinks that as you approach heaven, you first walk through some bushes and the bushes catch all the things that hinder you … all the illness and disease and other stuff. He said, "You walk through the bushes and then, POOF, you're Arnold Schwarzenegger." I knew what he meant, but still I said, "Arnold Schwarzenegger?"

He said, "Not Arnold Schwarzenegger, but someone like him … someone svelte."

I said, "You mean like a new man?"

He said, "Yes!" He hopped back on his bike and said he was going to do a few more laps and he rode off into the sun.

Molly and I headed home and Mike came home a little while

after. He did seven more laps (10K altogether) and "POOF" he was a new man!

I'm Not Giving You the Finger—November 14, 2011

I'm guessing we will never really adjust to Mike's illness. There isn't enough time to adjust. When we almost get used to one change, other changes happen. Day to day the changes are pretty subtle, but over time, they become quite significant. For instance, Mike was running six-minute miles in April and now he is just thankful he can walk ... even if it's only at a snail's pace.

Just over a month ago, Mike got a brace for his right hand. It's a brace he wears at night to prevent his hand from curling up into a tight fist while he sleeps. Mike calls the brace the "claw." While I put the claw on Mike before bed, I usually have a little pep talk with his fingers. As I struggle to lay them out straight, I tell them that, even though they are very stubborn, we still love them. I kiss them good night so they know they are loved and perhaps a kiss will make them all better .. it always works with Leah.

Today, we were getting ready for our ride on the dike, but, because it was so cold and because it was later in the afternoon, we decided just to go to Merkley Park again. I bundled up and then helped Mike put his gloves on ... not an easy task. It took a while to get each finger in the right hole and hold them straight enough to pull each one through. I talked to the fingers one at a time as I tried to put each of them in their proper place. "You are a little rebellious; you just need to straighten out a little," I said to one. "Come on, you can do it," I said to another. I really had to be firm with the middle finger. "Give me that finger," I said to Mike.

He said, "I'm not giving you the finger." I think Mike was enjoying the entertainment.

Mike's ability to cope with the changes continues to amaze me every day. He never complains; he rarely gets frustrated; he just rolls with the punches. I think the changes have been easier for him to take than for the rest of us.

In a message she sent me last night, Erin said she was really missing her dad. She said she was worried about him and hates being away from him. This morning she said, "I am feeling better now. I had a good cry last night ... and this morning ... and likely, I'll be getting one in at lunchtime as well. I wish I could hold myself together. I read an article on the bus this morning about assisted suicide and an ALS woman trying to make it legal and I broke down in tears. Luckily, there was a homeless man sitting beside me who gave me a shoulder to cry on ... well I guess not literally, but he did offer me some of his bottles."

Mike and I are going out to UBC tomorrow to see Erin. She can't wait to see her dad and I know when she does she will be encouraged. He has a way of making us all feel better. I think while we are out, I will shop for some mitts for Mike ... forget the gloves.

A Man on a Mission—November 16, 2011

My dad showed up yesterday morning just as Mike and I were getting into the van to leave to see Erin. He said he had called, but no one answered. I did hear the phone ring a little earlier, but my hands were tied. My dad, a man on a mission, took a chance that we were home and drove over anyway. He knew we were going to Erin's and wanted to give us a little cash to pass on to her for groceries or whatever. He also wanted the receipt for the new stationary bike we bought for Mike. He said he and my mom wanted to buy Mike a bike, but we beat them to the punch, so they insisted on reimbursing us.

My mom and dad are missionaries. Whether they are off feeding orphans in Africa, helping out in churches in Rio De Janeiro, visiting the sick here at Ridge Meadows Hospital, or driving a recently widowed friend to Port Hardy, BC to visit family, they are always "On a Mission." My parents started their charitable organization called Amazon Evangelism years ago and focused most of their work in Brazil. Project Wellness, a division of Amazon Evangelism came a little later, and focuses on caring for the needs of orphans in Africa—food, water, education, medicine, etc.

Recent articles in two local newspapers featured my dad and his latest trip to Malawi, Africa (my dad has done the last few trips solo). *The Maple Ridge News*, calling their article, "Maple Ridge Charity Builds Better Life in Malawi," informed its readers that Project Wellness drilled its twentieth well in Malawi last month. Twenty wells provide twenty thousand people with clean water, which changes those twenty thousand lives forever. The article also mentioned the schools built and the land bought for farming. It also informed its readers that all monies raised go directly to the missionary work and the needs of others. There are no paid staff members. All workers involved are volunteers, including my mom and dad. The only payment my dad has received lately for his missionary work came from a couple of extremely grateful Malawian women: two chickens and a bowl of rice flour.

When my dad returned home from his last trip a few weeks ago, he and my mom came out to the rink to watch Madison play hockey. Because I am the team's safety person, I am on the bench with the team during games, so in between periods during the ice cleaning, I went over to say hi and hear about his trip … I wanted details. He said the trip went well and without much further ado, he pulled out a piece of paper from his pocket. I recognized right away that it was a page from the book he reads every day called *My Daily Bread*. He said he pulled out the page for me because he knew I'd appreciate it. I read it and he was right. When I got home, I put it between the pages of one of my own daily readers, *My Upmost for His Highest*.

I've pulled it out a few times to read its comforting words. The writer, David McCasland calls the piece, "He Guards Me Well" and includes a beautiful paraphrase of Psalm 23:

"The Lord my Shepherd guards me well,
and all my wants are fed:
Amid green pastures made to lie, beside still waters led.
My careworn soul grows strong and whole
when God's true path I tread.
Though I should walk in darkest ways,
through valleys like the grave,
No evil shall I ever fear; your presence makes me brave.
On my behalf Your rod and staff assure me You will save."

McCasland goes on to say; "No matter what you're facing today, Jesus knows your name, He knows the danger, and He will not leave your side. You can say with confidence: The Lord my Shepherd guards me well."

At the rink that day, I wanted to hear about the newly drilled wells, the beautiful orphan children, the travel experiences, the adventure, the dangers, and so on. That would all come in time; but my dad, a man on a mission, wanted to quickly bring the focus back to the Shepherd and remind me that whatever our circumstances, He guards us well!

~ ~ ~ ~ ~ ~ ~

When your circumstances reveal to you that you aren't as strong and powerful as you thought you were; that you are actually very weak and powerless, sorrow floods your soul. The only thing you can do is completely rely on God, which is what He wanted you to do all along. When you completely rely on God, you get to know Him as the Shepherd of your life who guards you well and the joy is indescribable!

Chapter 5
Pride and Joy

I've thought about it for over three years and the only thing I can come up with is "pride" ... there is no other explanation. Pride in my life—in our lives—is what has made it so hard to receive, to accept gifts and help from others.

Letting go of pride is extremely challenging, especially when you are really proud like me and Mike. I'm not talking about the pride you have when your child brings home a good report card or scores the winning goal. I'm talking about the pride that shifts confidence from God to self. It's the opposite of humility ... it "comes before a fall."

Telling people you don't need their money, their gifts, their meals, their help sounds unselfish at first, but when you take a closer look, it's very selfish! It makes you sound like you are strong, but I now believe it's a sign of weakness.

When Mike was diagnosed with ALS, friends and family began to rally right away. The offers of help and all the giving were overwhelming. Mike and I were more "givers" than "receivers." We never really needed much help and we certainly never needed any "handouts." If we saw a need somewhere, we didn't hesitate to share from the abundance we had. Mike in particular was a very generous giver and still is. But ALS put us in a position to receive, and it was the most uncomfortable position we had ever been in.

Letting your pride get in the way of accepting something from someone, I've learned, is cruel. It thwarts thoughtfulness, it kills kindness, it slaps love in the face, and it obstructs joy. Most givers would agree, joy comes in giving and now I know it comes in receiving too.

For a guy taking good care of himself and his family, getting ALS is a big blow to the ego. Mike kept telling us it was certainly a humbling experience ... true humility is a hard lesson to learn.

We put a lot of importance in being self-reliant. We all have been programmed to "believe in ourselves"; it's called self-affirmation. While I think it's great to be confident and to believe I can do many things I set my mind to, I think it's actually harmful to believe in myself. Excessive belief in one's abilities interferes with God's power and grace, and it puts us in His place; on the throne of our lives where He belongs.

As uncomfortable as it was and still can be, we quickly learned to accept graciously. We are still learning how to let go of pride, but I will tell you this, there is freedom and joy on the other side of it!

What a Hoot—November 21, 2011

Ida from the Healing Room told Mike to look for signs that the Lord is near: to look for signs of His love. I believe there are signs all around us of God's love, such as oxygen, water, food, shelter, etc. But Ida was challenging Mike to look beyond the ordinary ... to look for the extraordinary signs.

Mike has a strong faith and he isn't the type of person who needs signs. He is already convinced of God's love, plus faith is about *not* seeing and *still* believing. Anyway, I knew what Ida meant. She meant that Mike should look for personal signs ... extraordinary signs for an extraordinary time in Mike's life.

The other night when it was time to go to Madison's hockey game, Madison headed out to the van with her equipment and Mike followed behind her. I told them I'd be right there; I just needed to grab a few things and turn out some lights. I was just heading out the door, and Mike was there on the front porch. He had come back to the house to ask me to get the camera. I knew right away that there had to be something extraordinary for Mike to be calling for the camera. I asked him what it was. I asked if it was a raccoon, because raccoons can be vicious and we probably shouldn't be getting up close to take a picture of a raccoon. Mike shushed me and said, "Just get the camera."

So I grabbed the camera and followed him outside. We went out to the driveway and he whispered, "Up there."

We both looked up at the owl sitting on a wire right over our driveway. Madison was like a statue. She said in a soft voice, "He's been staring at me the whole time."

I couldn't believe it was an owl. I have never seen an owl before, outside of a zoo, that is. It was a very large owl, and its eyes were in the back of his head, keeping a close watch on all of us. Owls, of course, don't have eyes in the backs of their heads, but they can turn their heads 270°. I took a few pictures, but I was unable to capture this magnificent animal because it was so dark. I do have a magnificent image of it in my mind though, and I can't stop thinking about that owl.

I've been talking about this owl a lot and Mike keeps saying, "Why do you give a HOOT?"

I wondered if it was one of the signs Ida was talking about, but I was stumped … what kind of sign was this owl? Maybe it wasn't so much a sign as it was a reminder. Maybe the Lord sent the owl to remind us that He has eyes in the back of His head. Well, not that He has eyes in the back of His head, but that He never loses sight of us.

Like never before, we find comfort in the fact that He never loses sight of us. This weekend on a road trip with Madison's hockey team, while we were about an hour from our destination of Prince George, Mike took his pills. I could tell there was a problem when he took the last one. It seemed like he was having trouble swallowing it.

I was just talking to him not long ago about how we need to

cut up or crush his pills and I should have implemented that plan right away. Mike was indeed having trouble swallowing the pill. He kept taking sips of water and looked like he was growing more and more concerned. He was breathing, so I remained calm and kept handing him the bottle of water and asking if he was okay. After a few minutes, I knew he wasn't okay. He struggled for quite a while and panicked a couple of times. Thankfully, one of the other hockey moms stepped in to help us. We were so relieved when Mike finally chucked most of it up, but small pieces remained in his throat for a few hours.

Later, he said it was the worst thing he has ever experienced. It was one of the worst things I have experienced as well. It was so hard to see Mike in that situation, and I couldn't help but wonder, with some fear and anxiety, what is yet to come.

As I anticipate what's ahead, I find so much comfort in knowing God never loses sight of us. We are not doing this on our own … He always sees us … He is always with us and I am not that afraid.

Meanwhile, I guess all my going on about owls has left Mike thinking about them too … I can hear him on the couch singing; "OWL be home for Christmas …"

Big Brothers—November 23, 2011

Mike's brother Gary was in town recently. He lives in Toronto and frequently comes to Vancouver on business. It is a great opportunity for us to see him.

Mike and Gary are eight years apart … Gary being the big brother. Because of the eight years and three sisters that separate them, Gary and Mike weren't necessarily that close growing up.

But they did share a closeness that Mike often speaks about—they shared a bedroom. Mike tells me that being the younger brother he had an earlier bedtime than Gary. He would have to go to bed alone and was afraid of the dark. He says he would lie frozen in his bed, scared of the monsters in the closet and was so relieved when it was time for his big brother to crawl into the bunk below him. Gary played The Beatles' *Abbey Road* record and Mike says he would fall asleep listening to what is still his favourite album. Mike's big brother offered something that was invaluable to him: comfort, security, and protection ... and some great tunes to help him drift off to sleep.

I always wanted a big brother. I have a big sister and, as a child, I dreamed of having a big brother as well. When my sister married her husband Peter twelve-and-a-half years ago (a significant number in Holland, where Peter is from, as it's halfway to twenty-five), my dream came true. I got the big brother I always wanted ... and it was well worth the wait.

Peter would do anything for me ... just like a big brother. Mike isn't much of a handyman, so Peter is my go-to guy. If I need something assembled, I call Peter. If I need shelving hung, I call Peter. Computer problem, leaky faucet, new light fixture ... I call Peter. He has put down flooring, put up a wall, and helped paint the outside of our house. He has shown up with his lawn mower (when ours wasn't working), weed eater, and that big saw-like thing to trim our high hedge. Peter is kind and thoughtful, and he looks out for me and my family ... just like a big brother.

Mike was lucky to have a big brother growing up and lucky to acquire three more over the years when his sisters got married. Like the big brother I acquired, his would do anything for him too. Big brother (in law) Mike is a fairly quiet person, with a large heart. A do-anything-for-you-at-the-drop-of-a-hat kind of a guy. I talked to big brother (in law) Ross on the phone the other day and just in the few minutes we talked, he said something that revealed his compassion and thoughtfulness. And then there is big brother (in law) Gary.

Mike and Gary have been great friends since they were teenagers. Their relationship reminds me of a verse in Proverbs that says: "There is a friend who sticks closer than a brother" … Gary is that kind of friend. He'd give you the shirt off his back!

It can get confusing because, out of five guys, there are two Garys and two Mikes and brothers-in-law Mike and Gary are brothers too.

On Gary's most recent business trip (back to Mike's brother, not brother-in-law), Nathan, Mike, and I picked him up at his hotel and went to a Greek restaurant close by. Mike had been there before and said it had good food and reasonable prices. He knew it was in the area, but not exactly sure where. We headed in the direction he thought it was, and sure enough, we drove right to it. Gary thought that was pretty good and said that he had a terrible sense of direction.

After we were seated, Gary told us a story to give us a better idea of just how bad he was with directions. He said that once while on holidays in the United States with his family, he and his three children ventured out in the RV. When it was time for them to make their way back to where they were staying, Gary got lost. He said he approached an intersection, and when he looked down the street to the right, he saw a fire truck, so he turned to follow the truck, thinking it was probably going in the direction of the town. When he heard the marching band behind him, he quickly realized he had joined a procession of floats, antique cars, and clowns ... he had driven right into a parade. In time with the beat of the drums behind him, Gary started waving and his three teenagers hit the floor. I don't really do the story justice, but when Gary told it, it was so funny ... we were killing ourselves laughing.

The parade story reminded me of something I once heard; something that has stuck with me for years, but I can't remember who said it. Anyway, it goes like this: our lives are like a parade. As we look on, we can only see one float go by at a time. But God, who looks down from above, can see the whole parade ... the beginning and the end at the same time. We don't know what tomorrow holds, but He does and that brings me a lot of comfort and peace.

Note to our big brothers: Thanks for everything! You are such nice guys and really great men!

My New Bike—November 24, 2011—by Mike Sands

Well, the verdict is in. Exercise is good for you. Those who have the get-up-and-go live longer, healthier lives than those couch potatoes who sit around doing nothing. Sitting around has repercussions for every part of the body. It appears the only thing that sat its way to success is a hen. Now I'm not saying that idle couch potatoes are not important to society. After all, it's lazy people who invented the wheel and the bicycle, because they didn't want to walk or carry things. With the onset of my illness, I knew it was time to get off the couch and get more active in order to stave off the symptoms. My only question was, "What mode of exercise would I choose?"

I joined a health club last year, spent three hundred bucks and didn't improve my fitness level one bit. Apparently, you have to show up. Recently, I tried aerobics, once. When I came home from the class, I told my wife I had to quit because I broke a toe.

She said, "How is it now?"

I said, "I don't know, you'll have to ask the lady whose foot I stepped on."

I then tried jogging. The trouble with jogging is that by the time you realize you're not in shape for it, it's too far to walk back. Cycling was the ideal fit for me. Cycling is low impact on the joints and it offers you a chance to enjoy a scenic view while getting healthy. I had a rough start to my fitness program, as my illness made it difficult to negotiate turns and my reflexes were suspect.

With the onset of winter, we purchased a stationary bike, which I've been riding for an average of ten miles a day. I believe exercise makes me feel better than any of the medication I am on and, therefore, will continue doing it until my legs will not permit it.

~ ~ ~ ~ ~ ~ ~

Right about this time, when Mike got an indoor stationary bike, his outdoor riding came to an end.

A Girl's Best Friend—November 27, 2011

Saying goodbye is so hard. I'm watching the final scene of the movie *Marley & Me*, where John, played by Owen Wilson, is saying goodbye to his beloved best friend Marley, a very old and very beautiful golden lab. I've seen the movie before and know that the ending is horribly sad, but I continue to watch it anyway, breaking my rule of NO SAD MOVIES! Watching that final scene reminds me of a scene in my own life where I had to say goodbye to my beloved friend Isla (pronounced like Island).

Isla was Madison's dog. Madison asked me every day from the day she could talk if she could get a dog, and 3,650 days later, I said yes. So, off to the dog pound we went to find the dog of Madison's dreams, which she thought was going to be a black lab. We went to a dog shelter about an hour away and saw seven black labs, but none of them fit the bill. I said to the lady at the shelter, "Look, we aren't going home without a dog!"

She sent us to another shelter in the area and there we fell in love with Isla, a German Shepherd Husky cross with one blue eye and one brown eye. Isla was already seven years old, but a puppy at heart. She fit right in with the family and was so grateful to be wanted.

Even though Isla developed terrible arthritis, she would chase a ball for hours. She was obedient and loyal, and she was beautiful on the inside and outside ... like most dogs. She grew old gracefully and toward the end, we dreaded the inevitable. I prayed that we wouldn't have to put her down; that she would go peacefully at home ... the way we all want to go. I was, however, not going to dig my heels in. If she was suffering, I would do what had to be done. I always said that as long as she eats and wags her tail, she isn't going anywhere.

A few days after Isla stopped eating and wagging her tail, I suggested to Mike we take her to have her put down. He insisted we give her the weekend to improve and if there were no improvements, we would take her. On Tuesday morning, Mike woke me up and said that Isla had taken a turn for the worse and he would come home from work at lunch and we would do what we dreaded doing. I got up and hurried out to the backyard where Isla was trying to get comfortable. I watched her take her last few steps and collapse on the dewy grass. I went and got a blanket and my Bible. I covered her with the blanket and sat down beside her. I opened my Bible to Psalm 1 and read out loud. The verses brought me comfort and the sound of my voice brought her comfort. The sun was shining and the birds were singing and our backyard became a little like heaven as Isla found her way to a better place. Just before she took her last breath, I read Psalm 46:10-11, which says: "Be still and know that I am God ... the Lord Almighty is with us; He is our fortress."

My friend Hilary who works at a veterinary hospital came with a co-worker and picked Isla up and as they drove off, I blew Isla one last kiss.

Today, our friend Celeste and her pretty five-year-old came by to say hi and give a gift and a beautiful card. On the front of the card, it says: "To everything there is a season. Ecclesiastes 3:1-2 says: 'There is a time for everything, and a season for every activity under heaven: a time to be born and a time to die ...'"

On that cool October morning two years ago, Isla's season of living came to an end. Isla lived life to the fullest and with gratitude ... a valuable lesson we can all learn from man's best friend and a girl's best friend.

Chapter 5

It Takes a Village—November 30, 2011

They say it takes a village to raise a child; I'm thinking it takes a village to support a guy with ALS.

Alan from "Jim's Mowing" came over yesterday to put up our Christmas lights. I wondered if Alan and his young assistant knew I was feeling a little blue, and decided to come by to cheer me up. They had no idea, but that's what happened when these two men showed up with a really tall ladder to hang our lights.

A few weeks ago, I opened the front door and a man was on the porch just about to put an envelope in our mailbox. He said hello and told me his name was Alan and handed me the envelope. He said he was from Jim's Mowing and that he saw the article about us called "Sands of Time" in the *Maple Ridge News*. He said he and his colleagues wanted to offer their services free of charge … raking, mowing, weeding, gutter cleaning, etc. I took the envelope and thanked him. I was at a loss for words and got a little choked up. I didn't even shake his hand … I just kind of stood there. Alan said he was impressed with our courage and genuinely wanted to help.

My mom was over at the time, so I opened the letter and read it out loud. The letter said that he—Alan—and a number of his colleagues in their organization read our story. He said that our fortitude and courage are a lesson to them all and they agreed a letter should be sent asking if there was anything they could do to help us. The letter stated that they had decided last year to try and support the ALS society and those who are coping with ALS, because one of their own guys is in a similar situation. He said they were not seeking publicity, recognition, or any gain, but just sincerely and honestly wanted to help. He said they very much hoped to hear from us. My mom and I both with tears in our eyes said, "Wow!" in unison.

I emailed Alan a few days later and thanked him very much for his thoughtfulness and generosity. I told him that perhaps in the springtime, he could do some yard work for us. He quickly responded and said, "Do you need your Christmas lights hung? How about your gutters cleaned?" What a guy ... what a great guy!

Alan is an answer to prayer. As Mike and I pray every day that the Lord will provide for our needs, He supplies faithfully!

P.S. Peter, my dad, our friend Ken, and Jim from next door help with outdoor (and sometimes indoor) projects. It was just nice not having to ask anyone!

It Takes a Village—Part 2—December 3, 2011

Since Mike's diagnosis, friends and family and people we don't even know have blessed us with cards, gifts, books, fruit baskets, money, flowers, food—including homemade pies and soups, messages of encouragement, and more.

In the summer, our friends and fellow hockey moms, Audrey and Karen hosted a BBQ in our honour at Gregg and Audrey's beautiful home. They invited the local hockey community and some other friends. Everyone brought food and there were games for the kids and beautiful gift baskets that our dear friend Adele put together and raffled off. We received cards of encouragement and donations that went to Mike's half-handicap fund.

A few days before the BBQ, a friend and another fellow hockey mom, Shonia pulled me aside after hockey practice and told me that every year, she and her husband Steve donate some money from their family business toward the teams their daughters play on … a type of sponsorship She said that this year, instead of giving it to the team, they took the money and paid Madison's first instalment for the season. I thanked her, and told her it wasn't necessary, because family had already given us money for the whole season and she said, "Well, it's paid for."

Mike and I have always believed that the Lord would provide for us … and He always has. But being very capable and hardworking, Mike would just pick up extra shifts if we had extra expenses. As of March 7, there haven't been any extra shifts, there aren't any shifts at all, so we have had to put our money where our mouth is and *really* trust the Lord … and He continues to supply faithfully.

> *"If God puts you into adversity, He is adequately sufficient*
> *to supply all your needs."*
> **Oswald Chambers from Philippians 4:19**

~ ~ ~ ~ ~ ~ ~

When Audrey told me about the BBQ fundraiser, I tried to talk her out of it. I told her not to worry about us, that we were going to be just fine. I told her that Mike had a nice long-term disability insurance plan and while it was quite a bit less than what Mike made, it certainly would get us by. She ignored what I said and went ahead with her plans. I remember explaining it to Elanna, telling her I didn't want people to think we were desperate or something. Elanna told me that people wanted to help and this was a way they could help in what seemed a desperate situation. She told me I had to let them do it. We learned we had to let go of our pride and accept the love and—you know what?—it's been an amazing journey of letting go of some things and receiving other things and experiencing joy.

Our village is incredible! It's concentrated in our community but spreads out over a great distance. There have been other fundraisers and many, many gifts. I couldn't blog about all of it. I did blog about some, including the "Summer for Sands" fundraiser at Fabulous Feet, a local dance studio. Debbie, Justina, Tammy, Adele, Kim, Linda, and others organized activities, dance productions, and draw prizes … It was incredible!

Friends from hockey and soccer and church and work … from the past and the present, and from near and far have continuously given—I keep thinking people are going to get tired of giving to us, but they don't … they tirelessly give! And of course more important than the money and gifts given is the overwhelming love and support of dear friends.

Not receiving graciously with gratitude stifles joy in the giver's life and it cuts off a multitude of blessings in your own life as a receiver. So now instead of arguing or trying to convince people we are okay, we just say, "Thank you!"

Chapter 6
In the Clouds

Tooth and Nail—December 6, 2011

My dear husband is hanging on to his independence tooth and nail. He reminded me the other day that he can still do the banking. I wanted to help him, but he insisted I wait for him in the car. I respected his wishes and from the driver's seat, I watched him slowly make his way into the bank. After some time, when I was just about to go check on him, he came out … with a smile on his face that said, "Banking accomplished!"

When I see him struggle with something, I jump in to help, only to hear him say, "I can do it." There are certain things he graciously allows me to do for him now, simply because his half handicap limits him. For instance, it's difficult for him to take off his sweaty socks after a bike ride, so I peel them off along with his sweaty T-shirt. Sometimes I help him on with his pants, sweatshirt, and jacket. I am constantly asking if he needs a snack, a drink, a sweater, a massage. I ask if he is too warm, too cold, tired, hungry, etc. I'm sure I bug him sometimes, but I can't stand the thought of him not being comfortable and not asking for help if he needs it.

I know it bothers him that he can't help bring in the groceries or change the 18-litre water jug on the water cooler any more. He used to like washing the kitchen floor, knowing I loved to come home and see it shine. The things most people complain about, like washing dishes, Mike misses being able to do. He would give anything to do a load of laundry, or change a light bulb, or wash a window, but those things are things of the past.

Mike is a fighter though, and he will fight to maintain the little independence he has left ... and the one-liners are still coming on strong.

I continue to watch Mike in amazement—his bravery, his humility, his patience, and his determination. Sometimes, I just stare at him. I examine the toll ALS has taken on his body, but his face is the same to me: the variety of wonderful expressions, the warmth of his smile, and the sparkle in his eyes.

There is something else that hasn't changed as well: his amazing attitude! Still not one complaint ... not one!

~ ~ ~ ~ ~ ~ ~

ALS With Courage is mostly a stay-positive-in-difficult-times story. The theme throughout is Mike's incredible determination and excellent attitude. But in amongst the amazing and profound lessons I was learning and writing about came a knot in my stomach—anxiety.

I've had one anxiety attack in my life and I had no idea what it was when it happened. It took place in 2003 in Nigeria, Africa, about a thousand feet in the air. My mom and dad and I had just begun our journey home from a seven-day stay in Benin City. We were there helping some churches with a citywide outreach event; my dad had been the main speaker.

We arrived a week earlier in Lagos, the main centre of Nigeria, and drove to our destination of Benin City—about an eight-hour drive on a road with huge potholes all along the way. The driver kept weaving from side to side trying to avoid the huge craters, with little success. The sights were interesting to say the least, but the weaving and the jarring was horrific!

Journalist, Adewale Giwa, wrote the following in an article in a Nigerian newspaper regarding the Lagos-Benin Road:

"The distance between Lagos and Benin City is about 250 km; if one drives at 100 km per hour, the journey can be covered in two and a half hours. That is, however, not possible due to the poor nature of the road; the journey can last a whole day. Indeed for years, the road has been a nightmare for travellers." Before recent repairs, Giwa says, "The route was regarded by many as 'a death trap' ... Apart from claiming hundreds of lives of Nigerians, the road has also been an abode for the men of the underworld who robbed unsuspecting travellers ..."

Need more be said? About ten minutes into the nightmarish road trip, we made the decision to fly back to Lagos when it was time to return.

The trip back by plane was nightmarish though as well. The thirty-seat twin engine flew low because, as I found out later, if necessary they would land the plane on the road, which they frequently did to make repairs.

The turbulence was so bad and I kept thinking when we get out of the clouds it will stop bouncing, but we never rose above the clouds, and the flight was worse than the road trip. Fear and illness came over me resulting in extreme anxiety.

I was doubled over in my seat and I remember continually quoting in my head some of the words from Zephaniah 3:17, the way I remembered it, "The Lord your God is with you, He is mighty to save. He will take great delight in you, He will quiet you with His love, He will rejoice over you with singing."

Those words and my mom's hand on my back, gently rubbing, saved me ... seriously; I felt like I was going to die. I had no idea what was happening. As far as anxiety goes, any anxiety I had ever known before was pretty mild. I don't stress much. I do feel anxious when flying, but I had no idea it could go this far. I always managed to keep it together like I do in most situations, so this little episode definitely threw me for a loop.

We laugh about it now—how my mom managed to console me and enjoy the in-flight snack at the same time, and how my dad, sitting across the aisle from us eagerly searched for a barf bag in the seat pocket in front of him and never did locate one. My dad says, "I'm trying to forget the nightmare, but we shouldn't call it that. God blessed us with a straight flight! It was the first and last time I got sick in the air." And he has been on close to a thousand flights.

I've never experienced an anxiety attack again, thankfully. But varying degrees of anxiety became a regular part of my life shortly after Mike was diagnosed with ALS. When reality hit, anxiety came along with it and my fairly carefree life completely changed. Not only was I watching my husband's health decline, I was now taking care of him and most of the responsibilities: banking, paying bills, car maintenance, house maintenance, endless paper work, lawyers, doctors, taxes, insurance, and so on …

He Holds Us Up—December 12, 2011

"Worry" should be a four-letter word … it is so nasty. I am not normally much of a worrier, but I must admit, lately worry has become an annoying pest … more like a monster that just won't leave me alone. I wake up and there it is. I get up and it follows me to the bathroom. I look in the mirror and it's staring me in the face. All day long, day after day … following me, taunting me, nagging me …

"Worry" defined by *Merriam-Webster* is "a troubled state of mind, anxiety, uneasiness, distress." It's horrible! Worry steals your joy, it interferes with peace, it ties up your stomach, it dictates your thoughts, it interrupts your sleep … it's an enemy to the human race!

John 14:27 says, "Peace I leave with you; My peace I give you. I do not give to you as the world gives. Do not let your hearts be troubled and do not be afraid."

Sometimes, that is easier said than done.

So, how do you prevent your heart from being troubled and afraid? Oswald Chambers says: "You don't know what you are going to do. The only thing you know is that God knows what He is doing. Continually examine your attitude toward God to see if you are willing to 'go out' in every area of your life trusting in God entirely ... Believe God is always the God you know Him to be when you are nearest to Him. Then think how unnecessary and disrespectful worry is! Let the attitude of your life be a continual willingness to 'go out' in dependence upon God, and your life will have a sacred and inexpressible charm about it that is very satisfying to Him."

We were in Regina this past week for a hockey tournament. We started our journey home last night at about 5:00 p.m. and after a number of delays, we made our connection in Calgary. Because it was a very long day and a very busy and exciting trip, Mike wasn't in his finest form at 11:30 p.m. when we finally landed in Calgary. He stiffened up and was unable to walk from Gate 40 (where we landed) to Gate 43 (where we had to catch the next flight).

The West Jet people noticed Mike struggling and called for some transportation. When they delivered us to Gate 43, another kind West Jet employee had a wheelchair ready for Mike to make the journey to the plane. We were the last to board and, because the front seats were empty, we were told to take those seats if we didn't want to go to our seats in row 19.

We sat down in the front row and right away Mike commented on the extra legroom and all I could think about was my new seat next to the window. I am not crazy about flying and for that reason, I always ask for an aisle seat, plus I get up to go to the washroom a lot. I think to myself, "I can probably hold it for the short jaunt from Calgary to Abbotsford; but what about this window?" I closed the shade and tried to distract myself by watching TV, pausing to say a little prayer and to picture God holding the plane up in the sky with His hand.

Mike fell asleep about ten minutes into the flight and about a half hour in, I became a little curious about what was on the other side of the window. When I lifted the shade, I lost my breath. The snowcapped Rocky Mountains were brilliant. The million stars in the sky were captivating and the slightly less-than-full moon was stunning. I thought to myself how my worry and fear almost kept me from experiencing this amazing view. Feeling foolish and somewhat convicted, I had a few words with the Creator of it all. I had to apologize as He reminded me that I am very small and that He is really big! And that He holds us up with His hand!

"Can any one of you by worrying
add a single hour to your life?"
Matthew 6:27

~ ~ ~ ~ ~ ~ ~

At certain times, it's been way too much for me. I've said to the Lord many times, "It's too much!" But it's never too much for Him and He's been with me the whole way ... just like He was with me in the clouds that day in Nigeria.

"Clouds are the sorrows, sufferings, or providential cir-
cumstances, within or without our personal lives, which
actually seem to contradict the sovereignty of God. Yet it is
through these very clouds that the Spirit of God is teaching
us how to walk by faith. If there were never any clouds in

our lives, we would have no faith. 'The clouds are the dust
of His feet' (Nahum 1:3). They are a sign that God is there."
Oswald Chambers

Bureaucratic Red Tapes—December 15, 2011—by Mike Sands

Once upon a time, the government had a vast scrapyard in the middle of the desert. A thought occurred to them that someone might steal from it at night, so they decided to hire a night watchman. Then they thought, "How does the night watchman know how to do his job without instruction?" So they created a planning committee—one person to write the instructions and one person to do time studies. Then they thought, "How do we know the night watchman is doing the tasks correctly?" So they hired a quality control department and hired two people—one to do the studies and one to write the reports. They then realized these employees needed to be paid so they created a timekeeper and a payroll officer. But then they thought, "Who will be accountable for all these people?" So they created an administrative section with an administrative officer, an assistant administrative officer, and a legal secretary. After a year of having this command service, they realized they were eighteen thousand dollars over budget, and decided they needed to make cutbacks. So they fired the night watchman.[2]

---

[2]Read on the internet—author unknown.

Government bureaucracies represent 48 percent of our Gross Domestic Product, and are under increasing pressure to be more cost-efficient. They are perceived to be less efficient than their private sector counterparts because they are not profit orientated and have exceptional job guarantee packages. Stories of people being on hold for extended times, red tape, and run-arounds are common. The biggest complaint from citizens is all the paperwork that these bureaucracies force you to fill out in order to obtain simple services such as a passport, licence, or title transfers. It's almost as though the bureaucrats have taken a course on making the paperwork as long and arduous as it is, so that they alone are able to comprehend it. A good example is the following statistic on the amount of words used: Pythagorean theorem—24 words; The Lord's Prayer—28 words; Archimedes' principle—67 words; The Ten Commandments—167 words; The Gettysburg Address—286; The Declaration of Independence—1300 words: The Constitution of the United States with all 33 amendments—7818 words; US regulations on the sale of cabbage—26,911 words.

I recently had a run-in with the bureaucratic system. I was sent forms to fill out for long-term disability. I filled out all relevant sections, leaving the "return to work" section that is reserved more for people who have a sore back and will likely have a future return date.

A bureaucrat called me and said I forgot to fill out the above section. I explained that this section was not relevant to my situation. End of conversation.

Not end of conversation. They told me that until I filled out these questions, I would not receive compensation. No problem, I said to myself, I'll fill out the paperwork and send it in.

Section 1: *Expected date of return:* "Tomorrow."

Section 2: *Alternative jobs you could do if unable to do current job:* "Movie critic."

Section 3: *List dependents:* "The Federal Government."

Section 4: *Check this box if you are blind* (This one wasn't on there, but it wouldn't have surprised me!) The only requirement was filling it out and they got what they wanted. It's too bad if they can't take a joke.

Keep Calm and Pray—December 27, 2011

Among the many wonderful gifts I received for Christmas this year was a bookmark that says: "Keep Calm and Pray." It comes from the famous quote: "Keep Calm and Carry On," which was a poster produced by the British Government in 1939 during the beginning of the Second World War, intended to raise the morale of the British public in the event of an invasion.

"Keep Calm and Pray" was a very timely message as I was nervously getting ready for the Christmas hockey tournament in Calgary. Mike had decided a while ago that he would sit this one out and enjoy the time at home with Erin and Nathan. Even though Erin was going to be home from UBC and my mom and sister said they would come by with meals, etc. and Nathan said he would be coming every day, I was so nervous to leave Mike.

Mike and I have systems; we have developed routines. I know what he needs without him necessarily having to say; plus he feels comfortable asking me to do certain things for him that he might not feel comfortable asking someone else to do. Needing his pants pulled up a bit, he says, "Give the right side of my pants a yank, would ya?" When Mike gets up to go to the washroom in the night, I am ready to put the covers back on him when he returns, and place his pillows back where he likes them—one he holds in his arms and one between his knees and I fluff the one he lies his head on.

Although I enjoyed the most wonderful Christmas ever, I was a bit of a nervous wreck the week leading up to Boxing Day—yesterday, the day Madison and I left for Calgary. But then I opened up that bookmark with those words "Keep Calm and Pray." It was a great reminder and even though I had been praying, I needed to stay calm and trust that Mike would be okay.

I love the city of Calgary in the winter. It's white, it's peaceful, and it's calm. Calm … just like me now. We still have four more nights to go, but I'm confident all will be well with Mike, especially after the message he sent me last night. This is it:

Calendar of events today:

1) went to Swiss Chalet with Nathan and Erin

2) found a dime in Shoppers Drug Mart

3) got a back massage from Erin while watching *Judge Judy*

4) no falls[3]

A good day indeed.

---

[3]Actually, he didn't capitalize any of the words in his message; my editor did that. She used to work for the government, too

Not So Great Without My Mate—January 2, 2012

Madison and I returned home from Calgary New Year's Eve morning and were happily greeted by Nathan and Mike. Mike was pleased to report that Erin took great care of him while we were gone and everything went well.

For weeks before we left, I had been anticipating being away from Mike. I was worried that something would happen, or that he would need help and no one would be there for him. Something I didn't anticipate was escaping ALS. I missed Mike right away, but I didn't miss ALS and I felt guilty and sad. I felt guilty, because I could escape ALS, but Mike couldn't and I felt sad for the same reason.

One afternoon, we had a few hours of free time, so I ventured out for a long walk. It was a beautiful, sunny day, so I headed to the Bow Valley Trail, which wasn't far from our hotel. It was a gorgeous walk and all I kept thinking about was how Mike would love this walk.

One of our favourite pastimes is walking. We used to love going downtown Vancouver and just walking for hours—the streets or the sea wall, or both. We have walked trails and paths that lead to unknown places and many trails and paths we knew well. We have walked the dikes, around lakes, along beaches, and up mountains. We love to walk around our neighbourhood and other neighbourhoods and so on.

I was able to walk briskly along the Bow Valley Trail the other day, but would have enjoyed it much more with Mike at the snail's pace we now walk at together. I thought of the last walk Mike and I went on together; it was Christmas night and Mike was staggering more than usual. I held his arm and we walked through our neighbourhood looking at the Christmas lights. We went to the house around the corner that Erin has nicknamed "The Vegas House" and observed the thousands of lights like we had a few times before. There were cars coming and going and people standing along the black wrought iron fence, taking it all in.

Mike joked about how people were going to see us and say, "That poor woman has to help her drunk husband get home after way too much rum and eggnog."

I laughed and said that perhaps it looked like he was helping me ... that maybe I looked like the lush. Either way, neither of us had had anything to drink and I was guessing that the days of walking for hours around the City of Vancouver were gone. But I am not complaining. I will gladly stagger around our neighbourhood glued to Mike's side for as long as possible.

I enjoyed the Bow Valley Trail, but later that night in bed I quietly pleaded with the Lord that He not only extend our walking time together, but that He extend Mike's days on this planet and give him quality of life. May Mike enjoy the few things still left that he loves to do for a long, long time to come!

Needless to say, the great escape was not so great without my mate!

Faith Like a Child—January 9, 2012

I decided to ditch Madison's hockey practice this morning and go to church with Nathan and Leah ... it was a good decision. After some singing and announcements, the children were dismissed to their appropriate Sunday school classes. Leah got up right away and so did Nathan. They started to head to Leah's pre-school class and Leah reached out for my hand. The three of us headed to her preschool classroom with the other little darlings.

I have gone with Leah many times to the child-minding and stayed and played with her during the church service, but recently (even though she is still only two for a few more months) she has been going to the preschool class with the three- to five-year-olds. And she has stayed by herself a couple of times.

Today though, Leah wasn't going to let me go. Nathan left after a few minutes, but "Grandma" had to stay and that was okay by me. First we played in the spaceship, then we did some colouring. We watched some of the other children do some puzzles and play with the toys. Then it was time for the Sunday school lesson.

We gathered on the brightly coloured mats on a carpeted area in the middle of the room. We sang three short songs with actions. Then we sat cross-legged on the floor while the teacher gave the lesson. It was from Matthew 14:15-21—when Jesus feeds the five thousand.

"When Jesus arrived, and saw a large crowd, He had compassion on them and healed their sick. As evening approached, the disciples came to Him and said, 'This is a remote place, and it's already getting late. Send the crowds away, so they can go to the villages and buy themselves some food.'

"Jesus replied, 'They do not need to go away. You give them something to eat.'

"'We have here only five loaves of bread and two fish,' they answered.

"'Bring them here to me,' He said. And He directed the people to sit down on the grass. Taking the five loaves and the two fish and looking to heaven, he gave thanks and broke the loaves. Then He gave them to the disciples, and the disciples gave them to the people. They all ate and were satisfied and the disciples picked up twelve basketfuls of broken pieces that were left over. The number of those who ate was about five thousand men, besides women and children."

The teacher did a great job maintaining the attention of the two-and-a-half to five-year-olds, telling of the miracle Jesus performed that day in about three minutes. A story I love … a story that has reminded me over the years of the unlimited power of our Lord … and how He takes care of His listeners' needs. The children liked the story as well. Then they did a craft. I helped Leah glue her fishy crackers and bread sticks to the picture of the basket the children were given. Most of them just ate the fishy crackers.

After the church service was over, my sister who was also there commented on the really great sermon. For a second I thought, oh darn, I missed a good message, and then I thought, no, I got the message!

Hawaii Five-Old—January 16, 2012—by Mike Sands

I turn half a century today! Many people believe fifty is the age where we can consider ourselves on the "old" side (at least that's what many people younger than us may think). Mark Twain believed that we shouldn't worry too much about growing old. Twain's routine in the morning was to get up, look at the obituaries, and if he wasn't there, he would carry on as usual. My routine has changed over the years. Getting older takes its toll on the body. Not all your body parts are as cooperative as they used to be. "Getting a little action," now means I don't need to take any fibre today, and an "all-nighter" means not getting up to pee. You know you're getting older when your wife says, "Let's go upstairs and make love," and you say, "Pick one, I can't do both."

Your physical body isn't the only part to take its toll; your mind isn't as sharp either. As they say, three things begin to go when you get older—first, your memory goes, and I can't remember the other two.

Getting older has its upside as well. As we age, we become wiser. We have gathered knowledge and experience and turned it into wisdom and understanding. We always think of older people slowing down as a negative aspect, but in fact, it is positive. Older people are slower to respond not necessarily because their faculties have been dulled, but because they've learned that a quick response sometimes gets them into hot water. They're still playing with a full deck; they just take a bit longer to shuffle.

When I got up from bed on my fiftieth birthday today, I was determined to keep a fresh outlook on things, given the milestone day I face. As I came down the stairs in the morning someone asked me, "How do you feel?"

I said, "Like a newborn baby! No teeth, no hair, and I wet myself in the night." Not really. I still don't have a grey hair on my thinning head, I have at least thirty of my teeth still, and am I incontinent? Well, that Depends.

I still try to be young at heart, but it is difficult sometimes when you're around your kids as our generations are so disparate. Taking them through an antique store and saying,

"I remember these," doesn't help. Sometimes you feel like you were born on a different planet than them, as they have never experienced life without cable or a remote control, making popcorn anywhere other than in a microwave, using a bottle opener instead of having twist off pop bottles.

I've learned a lot in my half-century and will keep learning; just today on my fiftieth I learned that at twenty years old I worried what others thought of me. At thirty-five, I didn't care what they thought of me. Now today at fifty, I've discovered they hadn't been thinking of me at all.

It's important that when we get older we not lose the desire to keep learning; when we sit back and are content to just reminisce about the good old days, then that is a sign of old age. As well, we can't regret growing old as it is a privilege that many people do not experience.

Happy Bar Mitzvah, Leroy!—January 21, 2012

The most memorable birthday cake I ever had was a cake that Mike got me about twelve years ago that said, "Happy Bar Mitzvah Leroy." He said he couldn't pass up the really good deal he got on the cake that someone had ordered, but never picked up. So now, it's common in our family to hear "Happy Bar Mitzvah Leroy" on our birthday instead of the usual. I believed Mike's cake story for about a minute. I had been with him long enough to know he ordered the cake that way to see if he could get a rise out of me, but I just laughed … and so did everyone else.

I asked Mike about a week before his birthday how he felt about turning fifty and he said he felt good about it. He said he feels like he will have "made it" when he turns fifty.

It's funny because Mike had a thing about his age when we first met. I was nineteen and he was twenty-three when we got engaged. Then he told me he was really twenty-six. Had I known his real age when we met, I might not have dated him … I might have thought he was too old for me. I did wonder how he'd accomplished so much for a twenty-three year old though; grade thirteen, three years of university, two years in the army, a job as a forest ranger, a job as a life guard, some travelling, and so on. When he told me he was really twenty-six that made more sense.

Mike got over the age thing a while ago and when he was diagnosed with ALS in March, his fiftieth birthday became a desired milestone. He would say that if he could make it to fifty, he would be happy. He would also say that lots of people would have been happy to make it to fifty.

The couple of weeks leading up to Mike's birthday were filled with grief for me. I have come to realize the grieving process happens in stages, and as the illness progresses, the degree of difficulty accepting the changes increases … and grieving the losses comes with that. But January 16 was a day to celebrate! We had to take our eyes off what has been lost and focus on what has been given.

Mike has accomplished so much in the half century he's been here. He has also impacted the lives of so many people in a positive way and has been a huge blessing to me and countless others … the world is a better place because of my guy, Mike!

To Mike: Happy Bar Mitzvah, Leroy … and many more! May the Lord bless you and keep you!

P.S. Mike received many lovely gifts, cards, and messages for his birthday, including a card from my cousin Gail from

Steinbach, Manitoba. She put some cash in the card and told Mike to put it toward his new career as a movie critic. Mike got a kick out of that!

Sunk Without Him—February 4, 2012

Thursday night was the annual board meeting (AGM) for Amazon Evangelism/ Project Wellness. As Vice President, I am proud and humbled to sit among the board members and beside my dad, the President, at these meetings.

At the meeting last night, my dad told us about some of the accomplishments of the last year: six wells drilled, a new building used to feed and educate three hundred orphans, and some food for those orphans for the year. My dad paused to tell us a story of how on his last trip, seven children came to him led by a little girl who seemed to be the caretaker of the group—she was about eight or nine years old. She told my dad that they were on their own and homeless and asked if they could please be included with the other children. My dad told us that he of course said, "Of course" and "How could I say no?" And then he said to us, "The Lord always provides."

The story reminded me of one of our trips to Malawi, a few years before Mike's diagnosis. Mike spent a lot of time at the local hospital. He went to the hospital every morning, with or without the rest of us (on this particular trip it was me, Mike, my mom, Erin, and her friend Lauren).

Mike would first stop at the market and get as many tomatoes and bananas as he could carry, and then head over. He made sure that every patient and their family members got a piece or two of fruit and a vitamin. He would make as many trips to the market as needed. Most days he had our help, but some days, he did it on his own.

Mike worked tirelessly and inspired the rest of us to keep going back. Erin and Lauren would visit the children, and give out stickers and crayons and colouring books, and my mom and I visited with the adult patients.

My mom and I got to know a man named Amos who was suffering with pneumonia. On our first visit, I asked if we could pray for him and he kindly accepted. On our second visit, he said that our prayers were answered and he was feeling much better. On our third visit, we brought him a small book of Bible verses and asked if there was anything he needed. He told us he was being released in a day or two and didn't have bus fare to get home. He said he could also use a clean shirt and some food for the journey.

When we came the next day with Mike's whitest shirt, bus fare, and some granola bars and fruit, Amos was overjoyed. I asked him where the book we gave him was so I could put the money inside to keep it safe. He pulled back the covers and showed me the book he was holding close to his heart.

The next day, Amos was sitting up on the side of his bed, proudly wearing his new "Run a Mile for Mental Health" T-shirt and a smile from ear to ear. I said a prayer for him and we said our goodbyes.

Once in a while, I think about Amos and how a little bit of help went a long way for him. That's what it's been like for me and Mike lately, too. A little bit of help from a lot of people has gone a long way for us for sure. And like my dad said at the meeting, "The Lord always provides!"

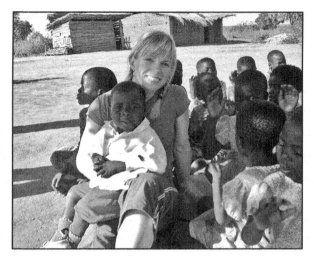

Nadine with five-year-old orphan boy,
Gerald, in Malawi, Africa

I have asked the Lord for help many times since Mike was diagnosed with ALS, and the Lord has been faithful and has provided help over and over again. He uses the people in our lives to help provide, and He always seems to know what we need just when we need it; not just for physical needs to be met, but for encouragement, reassurance, and hope, etc.

One night last week, my mom had to go to the hospital because she was experiencing chest pain. My sister and I visited with her while we waited in a room in emergency to hear what the doctor had to say about the tests that had been taken earlier. When the doctor came in, we were relieved right away. He was very upbeat and friendly and told us a joke. He and my mom had hit it off and she told him how much she liked him.

He assured us that my mom was okay and that she needed to keep an eye on her blood pressure, because it was a little high. My sister suggested that perhaps she was anxious about her son-in-law who has ALS. The doctor chatted with us for a while and I thought that was nice, because he had lots of other patients to see. Just as he was about to leave, my mom asked him if he was a praying man. He said he was. My mom asked him to please pray for Mike and me.

He put his hand on my shoulder and prayed. When he finished, we all agreed how much we need the Lord. The doctor said, "I'd be sunk without Him," and left the room.

Our niece Michaela who is almost eleven sent me a lovely message the other day. In part, it said: "With uncle's ALS, you guys show me how strong you are and how much faith you have in God. I know how hard it's been and I keep praying for you. I am willing to do whatever I can to help. You're always there for me and now it's time for me to help you."

"And without faith it is impossible to please God because anyone who comes to Him must believe that He exists and that He rewards those who earnestly seek Him."
Hebrews 11:6

~ ~ ~ ~ ~ ~ ~

After my anxiety attack in Nigeria, and after I realized what it was, I thought, "God will use this in my life someday."

"God can transform this destructive anxiety into a constructive thoughtfulness for the future."
Oswald Chambers

Chapter 7
Permanent Marker

When Nathan was fifteen, some of his friends were getting tattoos. I figured he was probably contemplating getting "inked" as well, so I did what any fast-thinking, concerned parent would do: I made him a deal.

I thought I could buy him some time to perhaps change his mind or at least spare him at that young age from getting a tattoo he might regret later. I can't help but think that when they age and their skin sags, many people will not appreciate their permanent artwork. But, hey, that's just me. I thought if he could wait until he was a little older, Nathan might get something he'd regret less … or not at all.

Anyway, just before his sixteenth birthday, I told Nathan that we would get him a drum set if he didn't get a tattoo … at least not until he was in his twenties. He took me up on the offer and I thought I was brilliant.

A few years later, while at a family reunion in Steinbach, Manitoba, when Nathan was just barely in his twenties, he had something to tell me. I was in the washroom of our motel room getting ready for the events of the day, including swimming, and I heard his voice on the other side, "Mom?"

"Yes, Nathan?"

"I just wanted to let you know now, before you see it at the pool—I have a tattoo on my chest."

It was one of those lump-in-the-throat moments. I was still really hoping he would spare his skin. My kids know how I feel about tattoos. I'm not a fan, although I've lightened up a little. All three of our kids have tattoos now; Nathan has a few.

The only tattoo on Nathan you can see when he is wearing short sleeves is one on the inside of his forearm. It's two words; "Let Go."

Thinking there was going to be some deep meaning in these words for our young man who is wise beyond his years, I asked him recently to please explain. He said, "Well, there's a scene in 'Fight Club' …"

Oh, of course, *Fight Club*—one of his favourite movies. He describes a scene that I wouldn't do justice to, but basically it's about letting go of control. A message that meant enough to him to get it permanently marked on his arm.

"If you seek to save your life, you will lose it. But if you will just surrender and just lose your life—for God's sake you will find it."
T.D. Jakes (from Matthew 10:39)

Faith Unshaken—February 9, 2012

When I came home from my class this morning, I found Mike out in the garage on his stationary bike. He assured me he didn't need my help when he was finished like he had needed the few times before. He told me to go in the house and he would come when he was finished his ride. I nervously agreed.

I watched for him to come out of the garage from the kitchen window. I was relieved when I saw the garage door open and Mike walk out. Steam was coming off his body and he was dripping with sweat, which is normal. He slowly made his way toward the back steps and I went out and met him there and offered him a hand. With a big smile on his face, he told me again he was fine and didn't need any help.

Mike was happy to report that he rode ten miles on his bike … he hasn't gone ten miles for about a month. It was obvious he was pleased with his accomplishment, and I was very impressed. Not only did he ride ten miles, but he walked down the back stairs, across the yard, into the garage, got on his bike, did the ten, got off his bike, made his way back across the yard, up the stairs, and into the house … all by himself. Then, he went upstairs to the bathroom and had a shower. The only thing he asked me to do was dry his back.

Most days lately, I have helped him out the back door, down the stairs, across the yard, into the garage, on the bike, off the bike, out of the garage, back across the yard, up the stairs, in the house, up the stairs to the bathroom, and into the shower. How did he know he didn't need my help today? Because he tried! Sometimes he tries, and is unsuccessful, but Mike just doesn't stop trying ... he has amazing determination. Many of us would have thrown in the towel by now, but Mike uses the towel to wipe up the sweat.

Mike is teaching me about perseverance, patience and the power of positive thinking. He has also taught me about a faith not easily shaken and about relying on God.

"Continuous, unflagging effort, persistence and determination will win. Let not the man be discouraged who has these."
James Whitcomb Riley

~ ~ ~ ~ ~ ~ ~

Mike yielded to God, and surrendered to his journey with ALS, but he didn't readily surrender to the obstacles.

"God is ready to assume full responsibility for the life wholly yielded to Him."
Andrew Murray

You Had Me at "Adorable"—February 15, 2012

Mike isn't your typical romantic. He has his own way of showing his romantic side. Mike and I have had twenty-five Valentine's Days together, but haven't really celebrated any of them. He did hit the ball out of the park on the first one though … he sent me *and* my mom roses. My dad was away and I guess Mike didn't want my mom to be left out. Can you imagine? I thought I was dating Romeo … until the next Valentine's Day that is.

Like I said, Mike isn't your typical romantic. He doesn't really go for the commercialism of romance and love. He thinks giving me flowers on February 13 or on February 15 is much more special, because everybody gets flowers on the fourteenth. There was that one other Valentine's Day that he gave me a beautiful gift, but it wasn't because of Valentine's Day—it was because I gave birth to our third child, Madison.

Mike doesn't buy cards; he has made a few pretty good ones though. Candlelit dinners aren't really his thing either. The lack of lighting makes it difficult for him to see what I have left on my plate for him to help himself to. He sometimes gives me chocolate, but not necessarily for anything special. I happen to really like chocolate and you know what they say, "Happy wife, happy life."

Anyway, this is how Mike swept me off my feet in his romantic way: He lived in a big house with a bunch of guys; the house was appropriately called "the Shack." I met Mike at the Shack when I was there hanging out with some friends visiting a mutual guy friend who'd just moved in; people were coming and going all the time. I had met Mike briefly a couple of times, but the third time's a charm and that's when we struck up a conversation.

It was the day before Halloween and I was telling him how I had to wear a costume to work the next day. I told him I thought I would dress up as a mouse, because I was a hostess at a restaurant and it would be easy to move around in basic black pants and a black top. I would just have to throw on some ears and paint some whiskers on my face. He told me to come over before I went to work, because he wanted to see my costume.

The next day, I was running a little late, so I didn't make it over to the Shack before my shift, but I did go over after work for the Halloween party. Mike wasn't there when I got there, but he did come home a little later. He told me he got called into work and not knowing I didn't come over before my shift, he asked me if I got the note he left with one of his roommates to give me. I said, "What note?"

He said, "Never mind."

I promptly found the roommate with the note and asked if I could please have it. He handed me a little box with a note. The note said something like this: "Sorry I couldn't be here to see you in your mouse costume before you went to work, but I got called into work myself. I'm sure you look adorable. Have a good day at work and Happy Halloween! Mike." I read the note and then opened the little gift-wrapped box. Inside—a piece of cheese! Well, he had me at "adorable"; the cheese just clinched the deal and the rest is history!

Okay, so it's February 15 ... my flowers should be arriving anytime now, but it doesn't matter because every day is Valentine's Day around here ... there is lots of love, that's for sure!

An Elbow in the Rib, A Knee in the Thigh—
February 24, 2012

When we moved into our house seven years ago, Mike and I had to downsize from a queen-size bed to a double. It was well worth the sacrifice to move into the home I'd admired since I was a young girl. This old house is in the neighbourhood I grew up in. My friends and I would ride by it on our bikes on our way to our softball games. We would walk by on our way up town, and when we got older, we would drive by it on our way home from school.

It's a small house, but a really cute one. The master bedroom is pretty tiny. I'm not so sure of the square footage, but it's so small I can touch every wall from the bed. I can close the door from the bed. I can reach my hand lotion on my dresser from my bed. And with the window at the head of the bed, I can easily close and open it anytime throughout the night. Mike and I like a cold room and a warm bed, so we sleep with the window open and a big, heavy, thick blanket … it's cozy.

I often call our bedroom a nest. It's like a hideaway … a little place of refuge. The Lord's presence is great there, perhaps it's because lots of prayer happens there. It's a place to escape. It's a place to hide, a place to read, a place to cry. It's a place we laugh and talk and cuddle and other stuff. And of course, it's a place to sleep.

Sleeping in a double bed brings you closer to your mate … literally. When Mike turns over in the night, I'm the first to know. I help him sort out the blanket and pillows. When one of us gets up to go to the bathroom, it's hard to keep it from the other. Coughing, sneezing, bad breath … just breathing and the other one knows about it. You can't not touch when sleeping together in that small bed. Mike's claw (hand brace) digs into my back. My cold feet find warmth on his. An elbow in the rib, a knee in the thigh, but we don't mind, it's a reminder the other one is there.

Last night was different. We slept in a king-size bed in the hotel we are staying at while on our last hockey road trip. It was really weird. Mike was way over there and I felt a little lost. Granted I had a good sleep … I stretched right out. I didn't hear him when he got up to go to the bathroom. I did wake up when he came back though, which was good, because I could help him get back in. It's a comfy bed and we are sleeping in it again tonight, but I think I'll move over a little. I don't mind the claw digging into my back, because I know he's there.

Iron Will—March 1, 2012

Yesterday morning, I taught an intense but really fun step class. After class, I went to the changing room to wash up, change, and blow-dry my sweaty hair. I know that sounds gross, but I had another class later in the day, and if I washed my hair after every workout, I'd be styling and blow-drying all the time.

While I was in the changing room, a young woman came up to me and asked if she could ask me an "ab" question. I said, "Absolutely, fire away."

She asked me how she could lose her belly fat. She explained that she had had a C-section three years ago and was still struggling to lose the weight around her tummy. She lifted her shirt to "reveal the ugly fat," but in my opinion, it wasn't bad at all … a little extra skin we all get to keep along with the bundle of baby joy.

I showed her some exercises right there on the floor of the changing room and she told me about her current exercise routine. I talked about strengthening the transverse abdominal muscles using the exercise ball and how to increase core strength with planks, etc., and I assured her that she looked great and was on the right track with her cardio and strength training program. She thanked me and left and as she walked away, I wondered if she had any idea how beautiful she was ... who is going to notice the little roll around her waist when they are staring at her gorgeous face?

I thought about Mike and how he exercises in a desperate attempt to extend his life and maintain some independence. Most of us exercise to look good ... feeling good is just a bonus.

When I got home from the gym, Mike was just coming in from the garage where he rode ten miles again on his stationary bike. He told me he felt great and that he is still strong "cardiovascularly." With a smile, he also said that his legs were strong even though he can barely walk. He was happy about the ten he rode at level eight (out of ten). He said a few times he felt great.

Mike believes that a good diet and exercise are very important for his condition. He went to Toronto in January to visit his family for a couple of weeks. He had a great time, but didn't keep to his diet and exercise regimen, and when he got home, he couldn't walk without help ... he couldn't really do anything without help. We both were very alarmed at how quickly his health declined, but after a few weeks of being back on his schedule, he improved ... what a relief!

Mike attributes his ability to ride his bike to a strong cardiovascular system and strong legs. Which is true. However,

I attribute it more to his mental strength, an iron will, a positive attitude, and a desire to live … not just exist, but LIVE!

I am very privileged to watch and learn as Mike continues to display such courage and determination. It's a humbling experience, too. I have to admit, I am just like the woman in the changing room; I have complaints about my body and want to improve how I look … what woman doesn't? But I'm learning to be more appreciative of my health—my ability to move, to exercise, to walk and jog and run around the house with my granddaughter on my back while the dog chases us.

Thanks Mike for your compelling example and for doing what you can to be with us for as long as possible. I am so proud of you!

**Brother, Can You Spare a Dime?—March 3, 2012—
by Mike Sands**

The Bible states that the love of money is the root of all evil. Mark Twain says it's the LACK of money that is the root of all evil. Whichever view you favour, there is a consensus in our society that money is important. Money may not be the most important thing in life, but as motivational speaker Zig Ziglar states, "It's reasonably close to oxygen on the 'gotta have it' scale."

Money is appealing and we all desire to have it. We realize, as P.T. Barnum stated, "Money is a terrible master, but an excellent servant."

The question I pose is, "How far do we go to obtain this dirty, filthy currency?" Thirteen percent of all coins and 43 percent of all bills test positive for harmful bacteria and yet society (not including the Japanese who heat press all cash at 395° in all ATM machines) lovingly covets it close to our pockets and hearts.

There are countless stories of people demeaning themselves for the almighty dollar. The TV show *Survivor* is an excellent example of this, where contestants lie, cheat, demean, and debase themselves in order to win the game and the money.

Marrying someone for their money is not uncommon. There was a story of the woman who was berating her husband for the disproportionate value he brought to the household income. She yelled at him, "If it weren't for my money, this couch wouldn't be here. And if it wasn't for my money, this house wouldn't be here. And if it wasn't for my money, that car wouldn't be here!"

The husband then piped up, "Ya, and if it wasn't for your money, I wouldn't be here."

This brings me to my story of how far I went for the almighty dollar.

When I was eight or nine years old, I was in Graham's five and dime store with my mother in the Highland Creek Village. I overheard a little girl say to her mother, "Mum, I found a dime." I was far enough away that I'm sure they thought that I did not hear their conversation. I then said to my mum in a loud enough voice so the little girl and her mother would hear, "Mum, I lost my dime." I'd bought into Will Rogers' philosophy that it's morally wrong to let a sucker keep his money.

I saw out of the corner of my eye the girl's mother motion her to give me back "my lost" dime. I took the dime and probably bought a chocolate bar with it that I'm sure didn't taste as good as it usually did.

Since that day, and many family and friends can attest to it, I have found an unusually large amount of dimes wherever I go. I find them on walks, store floors, ice rinks, almost everywhere I go. One time I found a nickel in a schoolyard field while I was waiting for my daughter. I thought to myself, "What's this? A nickel!" Not a dime! I took another five or ten steps and found another nickel. Last week, I found a nickel in Zellers; the next day I found a nickel at the ice rink. Even when it's not a dime, it adds up to a dime.

I don't know if me finding dimes is a way for God to remind me of my dastardly deed, or if it's a reminder to keep my path straight; but it definitely has given me a different perspective on how I view the almighty dollar and how I acquire it.

Most people realize large amounts of money won't make them happy, but everyone wants the opportunity to find that out for themselves.

Take it from me, after that incident, I realized money is not so important that you sell your soul for it; it can, as they say, buy a fine dog, but cannot make him wag his tail.

~ ~ ~ ~ ~ ~ ~

I always told Mike that finding dimes is God's way of saying, "You are forgiven and remember, money should never be more important than your integrity."

Since Mike's "Can You Spare a Dime" blog post, family and friends often message us and say, "I found a dime today and thought of you, Mike." Elanna seems to find a lot of dimes now too. She sends me text messages with pictures of dimes she finds in various locations.

Erin and Madison each have matching tattoos of a dime on their lower legs. They had the idea around Father's Day after Mike was diagnosed … it's kind of a cute tribute to their dad and a meaningful symbol to them. The tattoo is larger than a real dime and the boat on it, called the *Bluenose*, stands out with the water and waves. The *Bluenose* is a famous Canadian fishing and racing schooner. She was first launched in Lunenburg, Nova Scotia in 1921.

"*Bluenose* came to symbolize Nova Scotia's prominence in the fishing and shipbuilding industries … The majestic image of the *Bluenose* has adorned the Canadian dime since 1937 and three postage stamps, as well as the Nova Scotia license plate," (bluenose.novascotia.ca/history).

I love how the tattoo artist of Erin and Madison's dime tattoos made the *Bluenose* and the water the object to admire and how he embellished the waves. It's symbolic to me: there will be waves—there will be storms in life and, like I say in a future blog post, "I'm going to cling to the One who even the winds and waters obey."

Let's Roll—March 8, 2012

Yesterday marked the one-year anniversary of Mike's ALS diagnosis. We didn't celebrate the occasion, the diagnosis or the illness of course, but we do believe there are many things to celebrate every day.

A few days ago, a big white truck pulled up in our driveway and right away I thought I must have forgotten that Big Brothers or the Diabetes Association was coming to pick up used household goods and clothing. Instead, a nice young man unloaded a wheelchair and bench for the shower. When he brought the items to the door, I said, "Wow, that was fast." And thanked him very much.

Mike said, "I guess it's true what they say. I must have ALS."

We had just been to see the ALS team at GF Strong the week

before and put in a request for a wheelchair and they suggested the bench for the shower. We also signed up for the ALS Society. We had heard so many great things about the ALS Society and quickly found out it was all true.

Lisa from the ALS Society sent an email to introduce herself and let us know of some upcoming events. She also called and left a friendly message, letting us know that she was available to answer any questions and would love to talk and get to know us. I called her back and we had a wonderful conversation. She started by saying that she reads our blog and that it has encouraged and inspired others with ALS. She went on to tell me about the support provided by the Society, the few thousand pieces of equipment that get lent out to those who need them, the programs and events, and other interesting information. She told me about the researchers all over the world who ultimately work as a team to find a cure for ALS, and how people have dedicated their lives to this good work. She excitedly told me that she didn't think they were that far off from finding a cure. I told her that we are very hopeful and pray every day for a cure.

Shortly after the wheelchair and shower bench arrived the other day, Mike sat down to eat his lunch. While he ate, I wheeled around a little in the wheelchair and commented a few times how it looked brand new. Madison was baking in the kitchen and as Mike ate his lunch, he entertained us with a few jokes. He was acting a little goofy, so we were laughing at him. At one point, he said, "Hey, you're making fun of a guy in a wheelchair." He wasn't quite *in* it yet.

Mike has resisted the whole wheelchair thing and, of course, I don't blame him. The guy is a stellar athlete; fit as a fiddle. Most of the time when you ask him how he's doing, he replies,

"Great, couldn't be better." So what does a guy like that need with a wheelchair? I broached the subject very gently a little while ago and told him that we could use it when we are in a hurry to get somewhere or when we are out for a walk and he needs a break. I told him we could take turns; I would push him for a while and then he could push me. He liked that idea.

Well, today was a beautiful day and Mike was itching to get outside, so he mentioned giving his new wheelchair a spin. I pushed the wheelchair out to the end of the driveway and as Mike got in, he said, "Let's roll." Sure enough, about ten minutes into the walk, he wanted out and told me to get in.

Mum's the Word—March 18, 2012

I had a very nice conversation with Mike's mum on the phone the day before yesterday. She had called in the morning and left a message while I was out teaching a fitness class. I called her back while Mike was in the garage on his bike. She was calling to check in on her son and I was happy to tell her he was doing well. We chatted for quite some time before Mike came in from his ride. I said goodbye to Sheila and handed Mike the phone.

I puttered in the kitchen and was happy to listen to Mike talk with his mum on the phone in the other room. The relationship between a mother and her son is very special ... a mom is the first woman a boy loves. Mike and his mum have a wonderful relationship and share an interest in many of the same things— old movies, politics, current events, history, religion, and so on. I have always liked listening to their conversations; they are interesting, educational, and often funny. Listening to their conversation on the phone is a little tricky, but it didn't matter what they were talking about, it just sounded good; so comfortable and so natural. Mike didn't have to repeat himself once, so even though some of Mike's words would have been hard to understand, I knew his mum understood and I thought, "That's just like a mum."

My mom and Mike also have a great relationship. After my mom got used to Mike's pranks, they really started to click. She has found the craziest things in her purse ... sugar packs and creamers from restaurants, rocks, empty candy wrappers and other garbage, nuts and bolts (not the snack), and other random objects. She also has the opposite problem with things going missing from her purse. She has looked everywhere for gloves that have disappeared along with shoes, her glasses, and so on. Mike is relentless and she is a really good sport. They joke all the time and laugh a lot. They bring out the kid in each other and it's been fun to watch over the years.

Mike is really lucky to have two mums/moms and he knows it. Two moms, equals twice the love, twice the attention, double the birthday money. Some people don't have one mom and he has two and so do I and we are incredibly grateful!

The following is my mom's contribution to the blog.

A Love-Filled Family—March 18, 2012—by Sheila Klassen

My husband George and I have been blessed with two wonderful daughters, their husbands, five grandchildren, and a great grandchild!

Mike and Nadine in their early years of marriage stayed with us while they were waiting to move into a new place. Mike was a creative cook and taught me how to tell if the spaghetti was ready. You just throw a string of it against the wall and if it sticks, it's done. I thought that was a good idea until he didn't bother to take a noodle off the wall one day. When I noticed it a few days later and pulled it off, the paint came off too.

We got to know Mike and his antics quickly and grew to like him very much. We thought he was pulling our leg when he told us that his parents' names were the same as ours—George and Sheila—but *that* story was true. When Mike introduced his parents to us, it was humorous: "Sheila this is George; George meet Sheila; George, this is George; Sheila, here's Sheila."

Mike's illness has not kept him down. He does as much as he can for himself even though Nadine and the children are at his side to help. Mike is an inspiration and draws strength from the love and encouragement of his family—his family and our family … we are one big family!

Mike and Nadine are a true example of love and marriage! They go together like a horse and carriage. If one is pulling, the other is right behind. We never hear a complaint from either one of them.

Roses are red, Violets are blue, Mike and Nadine, they stick like glue.

A Really Good Book—March 29, 2012

Mike and I finished reading the Book of Psalms in the Bible last night. For the last couple of months, every night after getting settled into bed, I have opened my Bible to the Book of Psalms and read aloud the words found in this ancient compilation of prayer and praise. It's been like a late night snack … a tasty morsel that feeds and satisfies the soul. It directs the thinking away from the fears and worries of this world to the greatness of God. It provides comfort and joy and hope in times of trouble.

I started reading the Bible in elementary school. In Catechism class, I learned my way around the Gospels (Matthew, Mark, Luke, and John), the first four books of the New Testament. It's a good place to start reading this great big book. I enjoy reading about the life and times of Jesus.

When I was a teenager, I made the decision to follow Jesus and I asked Him into my heart. My "religious" experience was entering into a relationship with the One I read about and was taught about as a young girl. Now, He was more than a wonder I read about in black ink on white pages; He became my friend, my Saviour, and the Lord of my life ... I simply opened the door of my heart and invited Him in ... He happened to be right there knocking.

As an older teenager, I would lie on my bedroom floor with this great big book and devour the New Testament, soaking up the writings of the Apostle Paul and James, Peter and John. The Psalms and Proverbs from the Old Testament also captivated me. I would underline and highlight words and sentences and paragraphs that spoke to me in profound ways.

Over time, the Books of Isaiah, Jeremiah, and Daniel got my attention and only in the last few years have I really come to appreciate other Old Testament writings. But through thick and thin, through the good and the bad, the Book of Psalms has always been there to comfort and encourage me ... just like it has been these last nights.

Stormie Omartian, the author of my favourite prayer books, including *The Power of a Praying Woman*, says this about the book of Psalms: "If you spend time reading and understanding these prayers and then take them and make them your own, you will find a more satisfying prayer life. Much more than that, you will find God Himself. Then you will be able to exult with the psalmist, *'Taste and see that the Lord is good; blessed is the one who takes refuge in Him.'* Psalm 34:8.

Our Neil—April 10, 2012

Mike and the kids and I speak a second language. Even though our children speak some French (Erin being fluent in French), that's not the language I'm talking about. I'm talking about "Sein" language. We are all huge fans of the TV show *Seinfeld*. I have been watching since the show premiered July 5, 1989.

Week after week, for eleven years I looked forward to curling up on the couch on Thursday nights to see what Jerry, George, Elaine, and Kramer were up to. Mike soon caught on and the same with the kids (when they got older … reruns). It doesn't matter how many times you see an episode, it's just as funny or funnier the second, third, or fifth time.

Almost everything in life can be related to a Seinfeld episode. For instance, the other day, Erin went to the doctor and he referred her to a dermatologist. I said to her that I would like to go to a dermatologist to have some of my moles looked at. Erin replied, "You could pull an 'Elaine' and come to my appointment with me." She was referring to the episode where Elaine's doctor notes in her file that she is "difficult." The news quickly spreads among the doctors of New York and none of the doctors in New York City will see her, so she goes to the doctor with Uncle Leo and pretends to be his personal nurse. She tries to tell the doctor about Uncle Leo's ailment (really her ailment) in order to get the prescription she needs.

There is also the episode where Jerry dates a dermatologist; he refers to her as "pimple popper MD" and foolishly says she isn't a real doctor because she doesn't save lives ... he forgot about skin cancer.

Recently, I peeled an orange and it was rotten. Mike quotes Jerry, "Fruit's a gamble."

Nathan was telling about a really great parking spot he got. He said he got a George Costanza spot. Then he said, "I hope no one jumps out the window and lands on my car."

Madison was in the washroom today and I just needed a little bit of toilet paper to wipe my nose. Madison says, "I can't spare a square." I said, "Just a ply ... all I need is a ply."

When we witness an embarrassing situation (someone else's embarrassing situation), we say, just like any of the four of them would say, "That's a shame." Other expressions include "Pretty boy, Jerry. And you want to be my latex salesman? You're living in the past, man. You gotta get out of the past. You know this is my busy time of year. Serenity now! You're way off, waaay off! From now on, when you take a chip—just take one dip and end it!"

Anyway, I have been thinking about one episode in particular lately. It's the episode where a beautiful woman mistakes George for her boyfriend. She says George looks just like her boyfriend, Neil. George, having a hard time believing a gorgeous woman like her would have a boyfriend that looks like him, becomes intrigued and wants to know more about Neil. He asks lots of questions about Neil and becomes fixated on Neil, losing his chance with the girl.

The reason I have been thinking about this episode lately is because Mike and I have a new friend named Neil and we have become a little intrigued with "our" Neil. Neil first contacted me on Facebook and asked if I was the one who had the *ALS With Courage* blog. He explained that he had PLS (Primary Lateral Sclerosis), not fatal, but an illness closely related to ALS, and he had many of the same symptoms Mike had. We started communicating via email and I quickly learned that Neil is a lot like Mike. He has a very positive attitude, he has a great sense of humour, and he has a strong faith in God.

Neil has been very encouraging and helpful. He has also been very informative. He told us about a medication that has helped him with his muscle twitching (fasciculation). The next time we saw Mike's specialist, we requested the medication. We have always called it "Neil's pill."

We have been communicating with Neil since November, but just met him and his wife Donna, who live on Vancouver Island, last Thursday. Neil emailed us quite some time ago to let us know they would be in town for Neil's neurologist appointment at GF Strong on April 5. Mike and I were so excited that they were coming. They came to our house after the appointment for our first face-to-face visit. We all agreed that it was like getting together with old friends.

When Neil told us they were coming, he said we would have some laughs at his and Mike's expense … and that we did. Neil told us of the time he fell and broke three ribs (that's not the funny part); we laughed when he told us he called Donna at work and told her not to worry, that the ambulance was on its way. We compared stories and had a great time … we had a few serious moments too and we prayed … and then they were off.

For the Seinfeld fans, it was a Festivus miracle! For the rest of us, their visit was such a blessing! Oh, and Neil and Donna are huge Seinfeld fans too!

~ ~ ~ ~ ~ ~ ~

Neil had PLS for about six years and then in September 2012, after he realized he was losing upper body strength, his doctor at GF Strong confirmed his PLS had transitioned to ALS. Donna says, "Even the ALS team was shocked. As they said, if it transitions, it usually happens in two to three years. We were pretty devastated, as we felt we'd dodged a bullet and now it was like we'd been shot!"

Neil and Donna have become good friends of ours. They probably have no idea how much they have encouraged us. It's nice to have others who can relate in the sorrows of this disease and in the joy of God's glory at the same time.

"I tell you the truth, those who listen to my message and believe in God who sent me have eternal life. They will never be condemned for their sins, but they have already passed from death into life.
John 5:24 New Living Translation (NLT).

While Jesus never had any tattoos, He does have permanent marker on His skin. When you yield to Him, your name enters eternity permanently and "Your name is 'engraved on the palms of His hands.'" (from Isaiah 49:16).

Chapter 8
New You

Granddad Needs a Band-Aid—April 16, 2012

Mike has had a few falls recently. Thankfully, none of them have been very serious. He had one fall coming out of the garage after a ride on his stationary bike. I had just opened the back door to go see if he needed any help and I saw his feet sticking out of the garage door.

He also had a fall in the bathroom not long ago. I heard a bang and a crash in the bathroom and ran to find Mike lying on the floor. He was crying this time, so I thought he had hurt himself. I asked him where it hurt and he said he was fine. I joined him on the floor and we both had a good cry. I later told Mike it was okay to have a good cry about it now and then ... he always keeps his chin up and I wanted to give him "permission" to let his chin down.

The most recent fall happened on Easter Day. All the kids were home and our granddaughter Leah was here too. I was upstairs and aware that Mike had finished his bike ride. I was just changing quickly and planned to head right out to the garage to offer Mike some help into the house. Instead of waiting for me, he decided to come in on his own. Normally that's okay, but the back gate was closed, so Mike thought he would walk around to the front and was going to cross the front yard and go in the front door. But our front yard is raised slightly and as Mike tried to come up the slope, he lost his balance and fell. I could hear him yell as I was just coming down the stairs. We all ran out to where Mike was lying on the driveway. He assured us that he was okay, and Nathan and I helped him up.

Mike had some scratches on his back and his elbow was bleeding. Leah was very concerned about her Granddad's elbow and insisted that we get a Band-Aid for him right away. We told Leah that Granddad needed to clean his wound first and then she could put a Band-Aid on his elbow.

Mike made his way up the stairs to have a shower and I followed him. As we slowly climbed, we listened to Leah express her concern for Granddad. She kept telling her dad that Granddad fell off his bike and needed a Band-Aid.

Throughout the day, Leah kept confirming with Mike, "You fell off your bike?" She told Mike that she fell off her new bike and she kept pulling up her pant leg to show Mike the Band-Aid that covered the sore on her knee. She looked at him with an empathetic look. She knew what it felt like to fall off a bike … it's really scary and it hurts.

Leah wasn't quite two when Mike was diagnosed. She is now three and has observed Mike's health decline over the past year. She knows something is up, but of course can't remember the big announcement that Granddad has ALS. She never asks about it, she just adjusts to the changes that are happening to Granddad.

Mike loved picking Leah up and carrying her around the yard and playing with her. Throwing her up in the air and catching her, holding her on his lap, and doing other things that granddads love to do with their grandchildren. Unfortunately, Mike can't do those things any more.

Leah doesn't ask Granddad to pick her up, because she knows he can't. Instead, she climbs up on the couch beside him and then steps over his legs with one foot and sits down on his lap.

She knows Granddad needs help, but never asks why. She

waits patiently for us to get him ready to go to the park or to the rink or wherever it is we are going.

A few weeks ago, we were heading out and I helped Mike on with his sweatshirt. Mike said he should go to the bathroom before we left. He slowly made his way to the bathroom. Nathan and I waited at the front door and Leah followed Granddad. She noticed that his sweatshirt was folded up a little at the back. She stopped him and with her little hand she gently pulled his sweatshirt down. I will never forget those little red fingernails on her little helpful hand as she patted the back of Mike's sweatshirt so it would lie flat.

It's interesting to watch Leah handle the changes that are happening to her Granddad. She has a certain understanding and a peace about it. We observe and learn from this wise and special little three-year-old.

We Needed a Good Laugh—April 18, 2012

I guess you could say yesterday was a bit of a sombre day for us. It was just one of those days … no reason in particular. There wasn't much joking, there wasn't much laughing.

It was a long day and Mike and I were really tired, but I decided to quickly check my email before we went to bed. I had a few messages, including one from Neil.

Mike was sitting beside me and we both read Neil's email together and had a great laugh. We laughed out loud and it was a wonderful way to end the day.

Here is what Neil said regarding my last post, "Granddad Needs a Band-Aid."

"Hey Friends,

"Saw your latest blog about the falls Mike has taken and guess what, brother and sister, I'm with you! Hee-hee! On our way to California, on the way to supper from our hotel, I took a fall and scraped my arm as Donna was valiantly trying to hold onto me; good luck on that, have you seen me? But, alas, down I went like I was shot. Then in the room itself, I tripped and smacked into the wall, but as always, my head broke the fall. Then, oh yes, there's more! When Donna and I were in San Diego today, we wanted to tour the aircraft carrier (my desire, seeing as my father served on one in the British Navy) and I was doing great I tell ya and Donna, yes I tell you this is her fault, she says, 'Hey, let's see what's in here.'

"'Okay,' I say and as we go in, Donna leading the way, I lost my footing going over the high threshold and lost my grip on the door jamb and down I go flat on my back, but my head cushioned the fall so no harm, no foul. Now, I'm just nursing my wounds with rum and coke … makes for ease of pain. That's my story guys, no Dora Band-Aids. I'm sure it would make the healing go faster, but what I find is there's no sin in falling down; it's not getting back up even if it takes a while, right Mike?"

Neil's message not only made us laugh a lot, but it's a comfort someone can relate … it's great for Mike to know he isn't the only one trying to stay upright.

Spring Has Sprung—April 25, 2012—by Mike Sands

Everyone has fallen in their life, even the most coordinated. We have tripped, stumbled, and bowled ourselves over. Then we get up, brush ourselves off, and proceed on our merry way.

One time, a receptionist/nurse rushed into the doctor's room and said, "Doctor, the man you just treated walked out the door, fell, and collapsed on the front steps. What should I do?"

"Turn him around," said the doctor, "So it looks like he was just coming in."

It is our natural instinct to laugh, or at least chuckle under our breath, at anyone taking an unforeseen spill. We can't help laughing; it's funny. We may say after, "I'm not laughing at you, I'm laughing with you." Or something to that affect, so the person won't get annoyed at us.

Charlie Chaplin honed in on this natural folly of ours and cashed in on it. Everyone has seen at least one of Chaplin's flicks that depict him taking a tumble. One Chaplin short I remember had Chaplin walking down the road looking at everything and everyone *except* the road in front of him. The camera then focused in on a banana peel in the near distance. The viewer was on the edge of his seat to see what he knew was coming. But Chaplin, the clever artist that he was, threw a wrench in the script. Just as he was about to step on the peel, he noticed it and took a step to the left of it—right into a manhole. He kept the element of surprise with an old gag, and still got a laugh.

The banana peel joke has been around since the early days of vaudeville, but the use of the banana peel as an injurious prop has its roots in reality. In the early 20th century, refrigeration and shipping speed made the banana the most popular fruit in the country. And in the age of anti-littering laws, the banana was eaten and the peel discarded wherever the eater was. The peels rotted and became quite slippery and thus dangerous to tread on. Banana peels were in fact responsible for a lot of accidents and injuries. The problem was so bad that urban sanitation systems were set up solely to combat the problem with the peel. "Horse shit" you say? Well, yes, that too was a factor in urban sanitation systems being created in that era, but we'll stick to the peel for now.

With the onset of ALS come many problems. One of them is falling down. ALS attacks the muscle groups of the body. Over three hundred muscles in your body work to allow you to stand and walk. With the weakening of these muscles, coupled with balance issues, falls are inevitable.

I've had my share of falls. My most recent fall was three days ago. I was standing by the front door, minding my own business, when I lost my balance and fell into the door. I couldn't catch myself with my arms, because they are too weak, so into the door I fell. My luck, there was a nail in it to hold a wreath and you guessed it, I hit the nail on the head, or is that the head on the nail?

I've resigned myself to the fact that I am going to fall, but I'm not going to take it lying down—sort of, because, as the Chinese proverb goes, "Failure is not falling down but refusing to get up."

Unforgettable—May 3, 2012

Madison had a soccer game the other night at Westview High School, which is fairly close to where we live. It was a nice evening, so Mike and I decided to walk. I should say, I walked and Mike got a first class tour of the neighbourhood in a comfortable chair on four wheels.

I went to Westview when it was a junior high school and then I went to Maple Ridge Secondary School for grades eleven and twelve. Maple Ridge Secondary is just down the road from us in the other direction.

As I have mentioned before, we live in the neighbourhood I grew up in, so I know my way around the area ... the short cuts, the hidden paths, the alternate routes. Mike always jokes and says, "Are you sure you know where we are going?" Or he'll say, "Can we get there from here?"

There are many memories from our house to Westview. We could go a number of ways and they would all bring back fond memories. I chose a route that is quiet and quick, because Mike doesn't want to miss a minute of the game. We had about thirty minutes, so I had to choose carefully.

We headed out toward 216th Street and crossed at the cross walk there. Instead of continuing on the busy 121st Street, we headed one block north and took a less-travelled road toward 214th Street. I lived on 214th when I was a kid, but way at the end of the street, quite a bit further north. My friends Debi, Lori, and I walked to and from our elementary school every day on 214th.

Once Mike and I got to 214th Street, we had three options. We could go left and hook back up to the busy 121st Street; we could hang a right and quick left and go past my pal Jennifer Kendall's old house; or we could go straight through on a narrow path for pedestrians only. We take the path. The path leads us to a short road that connects us to Laity Street. We have a few options from there, but it's getting close to game time, so we had to make it quick.

We could turn left and then take a right, which leads straight to the school. This is probably the quickest way . . . this is the street Jen, Mel, Kim, and I took to Kim's house for lunch at lunchtime. Instead, I veer a little right as we cross Laity and continue west toward Westview down Jodi Bronson's old street. Half way down, I stop to say hello to a dog that was out in his front yard with his owner. Mike told me we didn't have time to stop for a dog, but I knew we had plenty of time, because after we pass Jodi's house, the street winds around at the bottom of the hill taking us to a path that leads us right to the turf soccer field in behind Westview. Mike didn't know about this path and was relieved to get to the game on time. I had taken this path hundreds of times when I walked to and from school with my friends Colleen and Kathy ... how could I forget?

The streets, the houses, the paths, the friends, their faces, their names, the laughs, running the track at the school, playing softball on the ball diamond next to the track that no longer exists ... I haven't forgotten. It was many years ago, but could have been last week.

Mike's brother was in town on business yesterday. While we were getting ready to go see him, I asked Mike if he was excited to see Gary. Mike said he wanted to see his brother, but didn't want his brother to see him. He said he doesn't want anyone to remember him this way.

We had a really nice time with Gary, and he and Mike talked about old times and childhood memories. We laughed a lot and squeezed as much conversation as we could into the hour and a half we had together. Our visit with Gary reminded me of our walk to Westview ... lots of great memories.

I told Mike later that we all have been given a memory and I assured him that he will be remembered as the well postured, broad-shouldered fast runner, fast talker, quick witted, vibrant, smart, funny man that he was and still is on the inside.

This was tough because while the "old Mike" slipped further away, the "new Mike" was taking his place and the old Mike didn't like it. He of course was having to let go of who he was and trying to embrace who he was becoming. I can understand why he thought the old Mike would be forgotten, but not a chance! I kept telling him we would never forget the "old Mike" and we embrace the "new Mike" and all his amazing attributes.

I don't forget my "old mom" who is actually my young mom, the mom I knew when I was just a girl. I can still see her large brown curls and smell her fresh baked bread. She has small silver curls now and I don't think she has made bread for quite a while. The point is I won't forget the woman she was forty years ago and I won't forget the woman she is now.

I won't forget her smile, her laugh, her inner beauty, her kindness, and outward radiance. I will never forget her singing and how she danced around the house, and I won't forget sitting on her lap. I remember sitting on my dad's lap too. I won't forget his perfectly manicured lawn and garden, and how he took me to the SPCA and helped me pick out my very first cat, and I won't forget piling into the back of his old red truck with a bunch of friends to go for ice cream. I'll certainly never forget my "old" parents or my parents now.

Same with Mike … I'll never forget the old Mike or this very special new one. I make a point of saying almost daily, "Remember how you always … ?" Or, "Remember when you used to … ?" Or, I'll make a joke or repeat a quote and tell him, "That's what you would say."

Chapter 9
Faithful Street

A Room with Two Views—May 13, 2012

This blog post is a story about how Mike's birthday present was one of the best gifts I ever got, and how God's faithfulness remains the same—great!

I knew it was time to get away when I told off the lady at the bakery last week. I went in to buy some happy-face cookies for a young friend who'd just had surgery and when the "mean" lady greeted me with that inconvenienced look on her face again, I kind of let her have it ... in the most polite way possible, of course.

There are two ladies that work at the bakery and the kids call them the "nice" lady and the "mean" lady and unfortunately for the "mean" lady, I wasn't very nice that day. I have been buying the famous happy-face cookie since Erin could eat solids ... long before the mean lady ever worked there. And I guess I thought it was time to let her know that her attitude wasn't appreciated.

It's not what she says, it's how she says it. She tells me the cookies were just iced and if I want one or two of them, I can have them on a napkin. I tell her I want a dozen. She gives me a dirty look and proceeds to tell me with an annoyed tone in her voice that the faces will smudge if she stacks them. I ask if she can please put them in two boxes, one layer in each box. When she gave me another dirty look, that's when I lost it. I asked her if she was okay, if she was having a bad day, or if this is the way she treats all her customers. I proceeded to tear a few strips off her, while she put together two boxes of one dozen happy-face cookies ... six smiles in each box. And one big one on my face, after putting the mean lady in her place.

I was a little testy last week ... a little uptight ... perhaps edgy ... I guess you could say *overwhelmed*! Our trip to Victoria couldn't have come at a better time. For Mike's fiftieth birthday last January, Gary and Aileen gave him a gift for both of us—a two-night stay at the Empress Hotel in Victoria, on Vancouver Island ... one of our favourite places! The Island that is, not necessarily the Empress ... we had never stayed there before.

The first thing we did when we got to our room was check out the view. One window displays the Parliament Buildings and the other, the inner harbour. It was a room with two great views! After exploring the room a little, we headed outside. Our first destination was Barb's Place for Mike's favourite fish and chips at Fisherman's Wharf; he has been there many times with his mum and aunt. We took the ocean-view route there and the long way back. We walked for miles and ended up at Pagliacci's, another one of our favourite restaurants. It was too busy for us to go in with the wheelchair, so we kept walking and went back later, and it was still too busy. We decided to go to a movie and when it ended at 9:30 p.m., we ran to Pagliacci's to get there before they closed at 10:00 p.m. and Mike got the lasagne his stomach had been patiently waiting for.

The next day, it was off to Dallas Road to where the land meets the sea. The wind and the waves and the amazing ocean view were just what the doctor ordered. My problems always become so small when I'm at the ocean. God seems bigger and my troubles seem smaller and my worries seem to wash away. It was a little therapy for both of us, and as we walked and talked and took it all in, Mike reminded me again of the wise words of Abraham Lincoln: "And in the end, it's not the years in your life that count. It's the life in your years."

On our journey back to the Empress where we were meeting Mike's Aunt Aileen, we came across Faithful Street, and right away I thought of one of my favourite old hymns: "Great is Thy Faithfulness." It was one of the songs on the instrumental CD we listened to on our way to and from Victoria.

The last year has been very challenging to say the least and I don't expect the next year to be any easier, but God's faithfulness remains the same—great! He has provided for all our needs ... comfort, strength, hope, peace, joy, encouragement, and so on.

We had a very nice visit with Mike's Aunt Aileen over ice cream and a chocolate milkshake (for Mike). Mike and I stopped in at Rogers' Chocolates a few times. We enjoyed our room with two great views and slept with the curtains open so we could look at the Parliament Buildings all lit up in white lights. We took a stroll by Beacon Hill Drive Inn where Mike's uncle Kaye used to take all of us for ice cream—before he passed away. We had a picnic in a park in James Bay before heading back to the ferry. When we got to the ferry terminal, we soaked up the sun while we waited for our boat and enjoyed every minute of our getaway.

We had a great time and feel rested, energized, and relaxed. And I'm sure if I'm at the bakery any time soon, to pick up some of our favourite cookies, I'll be more patient with the mean lady. I'll be nice ... I'll put on a happy face and thank her for being careful not to smudge her perfectly iced cookies. Come to think of it, she's not really that mean.

~ ~ ~ ~ ~ ~ ~

That trip to Victoria was our last romantic weekend away. Mike and I have made a point of getting away for a night or two once or twice a year since our children were small. I'm so glad we made that a priority; it was good for our relationship and, of course, those weekends away produced many wonderful memories.

This trip to Victoria was of course extra special—we knew it would be our last one like it. It was tough though—we were adjusting to so many changes, including almost full reliance on the wheelchair. We considered cancelling the trip, because we knew it would be super challenging, but I'm really glad we didn't … we had so much fun!

My role as Mike's caregiver went to a whole new level on this trip. We were on the ferry heading to the island and Mike had to go to the washroom. I had helped Mike to the washroom many times already—at home and in other places. I would stand behind him and help support him with one arm wrapped around his waist; I'd pull his pants down with the other hand. While he would do his thing, I would continue to help hold him up with both arms tightly wrapped around him. When he needed to sit, I would help him down, and then I'd leave and come back when he was done, and help him up again.

This visit to the washroom on the ferry to Victoria was a little different than the other washroom visits we'd made together—Mike needed help wiping his butt (I knew it was just a matter of time). It's of course a sensitive subject, so I tried to be as casual as possible. With my face in a magazine in the corner of the spacious wheelchair accessible washroom, I mentioned that I could help him out if he needed it. I didn't mind, but I knew he would.

Mike had wiped his share of butts as a nurse and now it was his turn to get his butt wiped … not something he ever imagined. I told him I didn't think it was that big a deal. I said, as a mother I had wiped butt plenty of times, just smaller ones. I told him, "You've wiped one butt, you've wiped them all."

He humbly allowed me to wipe his butt that day and every

day from that point on. I'm sure it was a relief for him, but definitely a low point. I have wiped his butt hundreds of times since then, and think nothing of it, but when I think back to that first time, I feel sad for Mike, but I'm so impressed with how he handled it.

My role when Mike was diagnosed with ALS was instantly "caregiver." Many people took on different roles; it's just a natural occurrence at a time like this. Some people, the closest ones, take on multiple roles. Some cook, some clean, some encourage, some fundraise, and some pray, and some bring you your favourite treat when you're having a bad day ...

You Deserve a Break Today—May 19, 2012

Wednesday was a rough day. It wasn't necessarily a *bad* day: we had a roof over our heads, food in the cupboard, clean drinking water, and healthy kids, so it was far from bad; it just wasn't great. Mike was a little frustrated to say the least ... things just weren't going his way and we were discouraged.

We went to bed earlier than usual that night. We thought it was a good idea to end the day as soon as possible and try for something better in the morning. We were eager to go to sleep and put the day behind us, except we couldn't sleep so things just got worse. Mike was uncomfortable and his legs kept shaking (he has spastic legs). He tossed and turned all night and just one turn takes a lot of effort, so we were both exhausted and by about 4:00 a.m. I prayed for him again, and finally his legs stopped shaking and he fell into a deep sleep.

I got up early and quietly did some housework. I kept checking on Mike and was happy to see him lying in the same position every time I looked in. I wanted him to sleep as long as possible; he needed to recover from the day before and from the restless night.

When Madison got up and told me she was going to the gym, I asked her to please pick up a large chocolate shake from McDonald's for her dad on the way home.

A few months ago, when I noticed Mike was eating less, becoming tired mid-meal, and losing interest in his meals before he was full, I started buying him McDonald's chocolate shakes. I knew they were really high in calories (a large is 1,165 calories) and I knew they would be easy for him to drink, and I knew he loves milk shakes. I make him shakes too, and he sometimes gets one from DQ, but he really likes the ones from McDonald's best. We now go there for family outings, the kids sometimes bring him home a shake when they go out, and we swing by the drive-through after games or shopping or whatever.

When Mike woke up on Thursday morning, he was quiet and still discouraged. I sat in the bed with him and read to him and prayed. We eventually got up and made our way down the stairs. Just when we took the last step, Madison walked in with the large chocolate shake. When Mike saw the shake in her hands, his eyes lit up and the smile we hadn't seen for over twenty-four hours returned.

Every day Mike has a berry smoothie and a banana for breakfast, but "he deserved a break today," and a large chocolate shake from McDonald's was breakfast (along with the smoothie and banana). Before he put the straw to his lips, he told me this shake made up for the one he didn't have yesterday. I knew right away that he was already planning on having another one later. He did have one later that day, one that my mom brought over, and as we were leaving for Madison's soccer game in the evening, he asked if we were stopping for another one after the game.

He was pleased and quite proud of himself by the end of the day for setting a personal record—three large McDonald's chocolate shakes in one day.

Congratulations, Mike … that's quite an accomplishment!

Nice Pipes—May 27, 2012

I caught a glimpse of my flexed bicep out of the corner of my eye the other day and was shocked. I was helping Mike up off the couch and, like always, I bent my knees and went into a squat. I placed one arm behind him on his back and one arm in front for him to hold and lean on. Sometimes we count one, two, three, and then stand. When we stand, Mike leans forward and my arm supports a lot of his weight. This particular time, I glanced down and to the left and saw my flexed bicep … it looked huge.

I answered the door the other day and the first thing the young salesman said to me was, "Wow, you must work out." I do workout. I have been teaching group fitness classes for over twenty years and as a kid I was always active in sports. But, the muscles came before all that. I attribute them to my Mennonite genetics (I sometimes call them "field-plowing genes") from my dad's side; although my mom had nice pipes too (still does). I frequently asked her and my dad to "flex" for me when I was a kid.

The muscular build works well for me as a fitness instructor, but when I was a young girl, I hated it (I was chubby too … it wasn't all muscle). My calves were so big I was unable to wear the really cute zip-up boots all my friends wore. Same with my thighs and the latest designer jeans—there was no squeezing them in. Over the years, though, I have come to accept and appreciate my muscular frame and now, as the primary caregiver for my husband with ALS, it's a real blessing.

When I pop a wheelie with Mike in his wheelchair and manoeuvre it over or around obstacles or down steep hills, etc., I ask Mike, "Do you trust me?" And he says, "Do I have a choice?" When I pick him up from a fall or help him up off a chair or in and out of the bathtub, I tell him it's good he isn't a really large person. He tells me it's good that I am really strong.

I sure have a new appreciation for nurses, furniture movers, and drywall deliverers. I am lifting and supporting the weight of Mike many times a day and just hope that I am able to do that for a long time. My strength is of course limited and the more help Mike needs the more I rely on the strength of God, which is unlimited. I call upon the Lord many times throughout the day for strength ... physical strength, mental strength, and emotional strength as well.

II Corinthians 12:10 says: "For when I am weak, then I am strong." It doesn't make much sense at first glance, but at a closer look, it makes a lot of sense to me. I believe that when we can't rely on our own strength any more, and draw from the divine strength of God, we are very strong!

By the grace of God, I will take the best care of Mike that the Lord musters in me for as long as possible. And I will do the best job I can do with His help ...

"I can do all this through Him who gives me strength."
Philippians 4:13

Are We There Yet?—June 1, 2012

The stairs in our house are becoming more and more difficult for Mike. At the end of a long day, I help him off the couch and we make our way to the staircase. When we get there, I put his hands on the railing, uncurling each finger and placing them on the handrail, and then I lift one foot and put it on the first step. At this point, we quite often look at each other and laugh.

After having a good laugh, we look up ... way up. Our stairs are no longer the short staircase we have been running up and down for the past seven years. Mike refers to them as "the Grouse Grind."

The actual Grouse Grind Trail is located in North Vancouver, BC, at the Grouse Mountain ski resort. It is an extremely steep and mountainous trail that begins at the 300-metre-elevation and climbs to 1,100 metres over a distance of approximately 2.9 kilometres. It's commonly referred to as Mother Nature's Stairmaster.

The average time it takes to climb the Grind is an hour and a half. Mike and I have hiked it together once. His time was forty minutes and mine was forty-three. Mike always wanted to climb the Grind again. He was convinced he could easily shave a few minutes off his time with practice. He says there's a technique to climbing the steep hill.

Well, there is a technique to climbing our stairs now, too, slowly and carefully. I walk right behind him with one hand on the railing holding tight and one on his back, so he knows I've got his back.

Before taking his first step the other night, Mike said, "How many more steps have we got? Oh, wait, we haven't started yet."

A few steps up and he says, "What have we got ourselves into?" About half way up, he says, "Are we there yet?"

We climb the stairs together twice a day: once for a shower after Mike's bike ride and again at the end of the day to go to bed. Sometimes, I time us and it usually takes between five to six minutes to reach the top. The five-to six-minute journey to the upper level allows for some contemplation.

I think about Mike's determination and how I probably would have given up a long time ago. I admire his patience and mental strength, and humbly follow one slow step at a time. I examine the grain and the lines in the wood of our beautiful wooden stairs and handrail. I pray for protection and for the kind of patience Mike has.

Elanna and Peter have invited us to come and stay in their ground-level basement suite (it's actually their rec room/ family room area). It has a beautiful guest room, a bathroom, laundry, and a large living area. They say it's ready when we are. But Mike's not quite ready and with his strong will and determination, we will keep climbing those stairs for as long as possible. Plus, he is convinced he can shave a few minutes off his time with more practice.

Come to Me—June 15, 2012

I have been very busy lately and Mike and I haven't been spending as much time reading scripture and praying together, and that's probably why I have been feeling a little anxious and pretty exhausted. Yesterday, when I finally sat down with Mike to spend some time in devotion to the Lord, this is what we read in *My Utmost for His Highest* by Oswald Chambers: "The questions that truly matter in life are remarkably few, and they are all answered by these words—'Come to Me.' Our Lord's words are not, 'Do this, or don't do that,' but 'Come to Me.'"

Oswald Chambers is basing his teaching on Matthew 11:28-30, which says; "Come to Me, all you who are weary and burdened and I will give you rest. Take My yoke upon you and learn from Me, for I am gentle and humble in heart, and you will find rest for your souls. For My yoke is easy and My burden is light."

Oswald goes on to say: "The attitude necessary for you to come to Him is one where your will has made the determination to let go of everything and deliberately commit it all to Him."

A few weeks ago at church, the Pastor asked everyone to write down a need or needs that they wanted prayer for on the blank cards that were handed out. All the cards were put into a large glass jar at the front of the church and a few people prayed over the jar of cards, asking the Lord to meet all the needs. The need I wrote down on my card was "rest"; Mike wasn't there, so I wrote down "healing" for him.

Last night, after Mike was all tucked into bed, I went back to the books to have another look at the lesson of the day. As I continued to ponder the Matthew scripture, "Come to me all you who are weary, and I will give you rest," I contemplated my need for rest and realized I obviously hadn't "determined to let go of everything and commit it all to Him."

It's a simple solution to all our big problems and the small ones too … it's just difficult to do, sometimes. I felt convicted as I sat with my Heavenly Father and listened to the words He has spoken to me many times before. I started to pray and ask Him to forgive me for not fully relying on Him all the time.

He just had one thing to say in reply: "Come to me." I dropped everything and let go of everything as well and crawled in beside Mike and found some much-needed rest in the arms of my Heavenly Father.

I am still learning to let go and trust the Lord with all my heart. I am very thankful He is so patient!

I Like Mike—June 24, 2012

This morning, Mike and I stayed in bed a little longer than we usually do. We had the opportunity to sleep in and even though waking up at 8:00 a.m. wouldn't necessarily be considered sleeping in, it felt good to just lie there for a while. At about 9:00 a.m., Erin quietly knocked on our bedroom door and asked if she could come in. We told her to come in and she joined us on the bed, on Mike's side.

Once in a while, Erin joins us in our room on a weekend morning for a little visit before we all get up and start the day. Mike and I really enjoy it. Erin rubs Mike's head or shoulders or neck and does most of the talking.

Erin has always had a lot to say, but she doesn't talk a lot for the sake of talking, she has very clever ideas, legitimate concerns, and bright and witty comments about a host of topics. Today, she told us about some of the experiences of the last few days of her teaching practicum. She shared how she was going to miss her students and how great the teachers were that she worked with. She told us about the surprise party they had for her, and the presents and cards she received.

When Mike was diagnosed with ALS in March 2011, our children of course took it really hard. Erin being the oldest and the most expressive, took the news the hardest (outwardly), and became proactive about the cause right away. She learned of the annual ALS Walk at Mill Lake in Abbotsford that took place in June. Erin entered a team she called "Team I Like Mike" and started inviting people to join the team and began raising money for the cause right away.

Erin speaks of Mill Lake often. She talks about how it was her favourite place to go with her dad while she attended the University of the Fraser Valley. Mike would meet Erin after work and they would run a few laps around the lake, or they would walk the path and talk about current events, or the courses Erin was taking that they shared an interest in.

Last week, "Team I Like Mike" entered the Walk for ALS at Mill Lake for the second year. There was a great turnout considering the rainy weather. Friends and family came from all over, including some of Mike's family from Toronto. Our team raised four thousand dollars and seventy-four thousand dollars was raised for ALS overall. The funds raised go to research and support for the people with ALS in BC.

Maybe next year, we will be walking to celebrate the cure!

~ ~ ~ ~ ~ ~ ~

Our "I Like Mike Team" name came from Mike's campaign slogan. Mike ran for city council twice. His campaign signs and other election material said, "I Like Mike." The catchy slogan was inspired by Dwight D. Eisenhower, whose "I Like Ike" slogan helped him become the thirty-fourth president of the United States in 1952.

Mike didn't win either election he ran in (he refused to align himself with developers, other politicians, and citizens wanting to tell him how to act and think regarding local issues), but he did well and received many votes. He also received a lot of recognition from his involvement in the community and his many letters to the editor regarding hot topics in local news. Mike's writings and opinions were so well received that he was actually offered a column of his own. Because of a conflict of interest, he had to choose one or the other and he chose to keep his commitment to run the second time for council.

After all was said and done, we both agreed that perhaps he should have chosen the other, because, like they say, "The pen is mightier than the sword."

Divine Intervention—July 13, 2012

It was wonderful having Mike's family here from Toronto to participate in the ALS walk. Some of them stayed for one week (Aileen, Ross, Gary, and George), some for two (Pat and Sheila).

It was evident right off the bat that they all wanted to help out while they were here. They were looking for things to do for us. It didn't take long and the guys were busy with some home repairs, the girls were cooking, and they all were fussing over Mike ... it was great. They wouldn't let me do anything for them. I didn't cook a meal, I didn't drive anyone anywhere, I just enjoyed their company and delighted in watching them dote on Mike.

It was hard to say goodbye to the four that left after a week, and great to keep the other two for a little while longer.

Pat continued to take care of Mike and look out for her mum. She has a gift of caring for people and whatever Mike needed he got, including more of her home-cooked meals—shepherd's pie, mac and cheese, lasagne, and spaghetti sauce (our freezer is full ... I should say *half* full now).

I knew Pat and Sheila weren't going to let me do anything for them, and with Pat busy trying to take care of everyone, all I could do was pray that the Lord would meet *her* needs, whatever those needs might be. And this is how I believe the Lord answered that prayer the very next day.

Mike had his appointment with the ALS team at GF Strong and Pat came along. It worked out well, because this appointment only happens every three months. On our way to GF Strong, Pat mentioned how she had really hoped to go out to UBC while she was here. She explained that she had been following the ALS research of a Dr. Neil Cashman who did his research at the university. She and Aileen have spent hours most days since Mike was diagnosed investigating ALS.

When we got to GF Strong we had to wait, which is unusual. While we were chatting in the waiting area, Pat noticed Dr. Cashman's name on the list of doctors' names on the door of the ALS centre. She said she had no idea his office was at GF Strong. She said if she had known, maybe somehow she could have arranged to meet him while we were there. We discussed how the chances of a busy doctor and researcher being there and available when we were going to be there would be slim.

A minute or two later, a very pleasant looking man with silver hair came out of an office to greet a couple who were standing at the reception desk. Pat had her eye on this guy and after the group of three went back into the office, Pat said, "I'm pretty sure that's him!" She said she had seen his picture so many times on the research articles she has read on the internet, she should know him anywhere.

Her face lit up and I could tell that meeting this man would make her day. So I went and asked the receptionist if the pleasant looking man with the silver hair was in fact Dr. Cashman. She confirmed it was. I told the receptionist that my sister-in-law had been following his research and would love to meet him. I asked her if perhaps he had a few minutes to meet Pat during our three-hour appointment. She had a look at his schedule and said he did a little later.

While the physiotherapists were working with Mike, Pat and I snuck out of the examination room and went to see if Dr. Cashman was available. We could see his image through the tainted glass in his office and could tell he was alone. I asked someone working there if they could please knock on his door and ask him if he had a few minutes to meet Pat. Just then, Mike's doctor, Dr. Krieger approached me with some questions and Pat disappeared. She was off to meet the guy she had earlier said she wished she could meet (I love it when wishes come true).

When she returned, she was beaming, and I think she was walking on air as well. When our examination room cleared and while we waited to see the last person we were to see (the speech therapist), Pat was happy to tell us about her impromptu meeting with Dr. Cashman. She told us that he said he was feeling very positive about the results of the latest drug being tested. He said that the results will be public information in December 2012 and the drug itself will probably be available in the New Year. She told us about the rest of their conversation and about the hug he gave her and how nice he was.

In the five minutes they'd spent together, Pat's hope for her little brother had been renewed. That was all this concerned sister needed.

Later in the car on the way home, I told her that there was no way we could have made that meeting happen if we'd tried. I suggested that the Lord made all the arrangements behind our backs ... she smiled and agreed (I think she smiled all the way home). With excitement, we talked about it again and again for the rest of the week. Pat kept saying what a nice guy the doctor was and she called the meeting "a divine intervention." We agreed.

~ ~ ~ ~ ~ ~ ~

Aileen and Pat have taken on a few roles from near and far. They come and go and help in so many ways that sometimes it doesn't seem like they live four provinces away. Pat, a nurse, has been instrumental in Mike's care and in teaching me. Aileen books the flights, arranges rental cars, and does the driving. And when Mike's mum is along, she is in charge of Mike's head rubs.

One major role Aileen and Pat took on was researching everything they could about ALS ... everything about the illness, new drug tests, natural medicines, government funding for research, researchers, fundraisers, all the stats, and so on. I think they know more about ALS than most doctors and other healthcare professionals.

It's a role I could never have taken on, so I really appreciate their efforts ... it's hard work! It's a difficult and stressful role no doubt. I'm sure it leaves them feeling hopeless sometimes and helpless.

The following are recent thoughts from Aileen:

"Lately, I have been grappling with my anger about ALS and the lack of serious movement in curing the disease. I believe it is within our reach to find a cure and I also believe research has been held back for many reasons. So many questions go unanswered: why are drugs not being offered on a compassionate basis? Why is there incompetence in the research field? How much money is being given for research?

Why is ALS considered rare? Why can't they streamline the process of getting drugs to market for terminal illnesses? And why, oh why, can't they offer clinical trials to all those who are willing to give it a go? I think we have become lambs in this fight against ALS. We do walks and raise money and make commercials for research, and it's been years and years of this, instead of rising up as a community and demanding something be done at the government level."

In another message, Aileen writes to me: "ALS is viewed as a rare disease, because the number of people suffering does not reflect the numbers that have died. It kills quickly, so it doesn't look like a good prospect to pharmaceutical companies. Watch the documentary, How to Survive a Plague. It's on Netflix and I swear it leaves you thinking about how we should be fighting hard for a cure. (It's about the AIDS fight, but it demonstrates the power of activism.) This is serious; WE NEED A CURE NOW!"

I have joked before how Aileen and Pat could very well discover the cure for ALS one day … maybe not, but it's possible they will be involved in some way. Unfortunately, they probably won't see their little brother cured, but someone else's little brother will be.

Chapter 10
Home, Sweet Home

My anxiety hit an all-time high. There were so many things to take care of and so many things to let go of … I could barely keep up. It seemed like endless paper work … Power of Attorney and wills … doctors' calls and appointments and debt to deal with. I dissolved my limited company and had to redo three years of GST, because I had overpaid—Mike always dealt with Revenue Canada and stuff like that. Madison was graduating from high school and helping her decide where to go to university was tough. because I knew she didn't want to go away, but felt obligated to accept one of the generous scholarships she was offered. We had our house up for sale, but didn't want to let go of it, and then the stress of keeping it perfect for showings was huge. I was juggling many things, but unable to save my husband; I kept thinking he'd save me. We were pleading for healing, we were letting go of so much while holding on for dear life.

A Math Lesson I Understand—July 17, 2012

Madison graduated from high school last month. She's our baby, so this significant event in her life hugely impacts mine. My chicks are almost all out of the nest and it makes me sad. I'm happy for her, sad for me. I'm happy for her, because soon she will be off to Mount Royal University in Calgary, Alberta to start the next chapter of her life. She has been given an athletic scholarship that covers her tuition for five years.

Madison was approached by coaches and scouts from different universities this past year with varying scholarship offers to play hockey for their schools. Being the team trainer, I was with the team in the dressing room before, during ice cleans, and after games. This was advantageous when coaches and scouts came knocking on the dressing room doors. I was able to meet the coaches and ask questions and ultimately help Madison make her final decision.

Needless to say, Madison is a great hockey player; she is a gifted athlete. Athletics has always been a big part of our children's lives and they are all good at sports. They are all fast, coordinated, and team players. I think what makes them stand out as athletes though is their determination, commitment to train hard, listen to their coaches, and try their best.

Anyway, Madison has chosen a degree program at Mount Royal that is a combination of business and sports, and Math 12 is one of the required courses; but she didn't take Math 12 this year, so she is taking it in summer school.

Math was my worst subject; Mike's too, so our poor children never received any help from us in math—at any grade past (about) grade four. Madison was stressed out right away. She was worried and afraid that she would fail. She was questioning her decision about the program she had chosen, she was talking like she was a failure, and that was just the first week of the four-week course.

During the second week, there seemed to be a glimmer of hope. While she was studying her math one day after school, she told us how the teacher had said to the students that if they listened and tried their best, they would pass his class. Madison was listening, she was trying her best … it's like the simplest math equation; one plus one equals a pass.

I keep thinking about what the teacher said and wonder if his students perhaps learned more in that one lesson than they will in all the math lessons of school this summer. I think it's very wise and valuable advice we should all follow. Whether in sports, academics, work, relationships, or whatever; if we listen and try our best, surely we will succeed. It's a great lesson for Madison and every one of us!

~ ~ ~ ~ ~ ~ ~

Early on, during Madison's second year at Mount Royal, she made the difficult decision to come home. She just wasn't happy being away and there was a program she was interested in offered at our local community college. I mention it briefly in a later blog post.

What a Heal!—July 28, 2012

The word "incurable" is not in God's dictionary, so we decided to take it out of ours. We believe that God has the solution to every problem. God knows the cure for every illness and disease on the planet. We have been praying for God to reveal the solution ... the cure to ALS ... ever since Mike was diagnosed in March 2011.

The human body was created to heal itself if things are right. Obviously, things aren't right in Mike, so the idea is to make things right so his body will do what it was designed to do—heal, recover, repair. So, we enlisted the expertise and help of a local homeopath and health coach, and embarked on a naturopathic regimen a couple of weeks ago.

Our new health coach set Mike up right away with a collection of powders (green and grey and really green), drops, supplements, and a really gross breakfast: organic cottage cheese and flax oil. It's called the Budwig Protocol and is used commonly in the natural treatment of cancer. One of the main functions of the Budwig Prctocol is to reform the oxygen uptake of the cells and provide good fats, the ones desperately needed in neurodegenerative diseases. Most of the other stuff is for detoxification and chelating (the removal of heavy metals). He gets painted with stuff, he gets hooked up to stuff … it goes on all day. Mike also went gluten-free and dairy-free.

Last week, Mike had his blood analyzed. There was a lot going on and not in a good way. Our health coach told Mike not to be too discouraged. Mike told him he wasn't discouraged. He said he would be discouraged if they found nothing wrong, then there would be nothing to fix.

Today is the twelfth day, and I must say, "Wow." I don't think I could ever do this. Mike has proved himself again to be determined, courageous, and very strong.

When we decided to do this, we agreed that it would be worth it even for the slightest improvement; to blow his nose or feed himself or go to the washroom with a little privacy or roll over in bed … to shake a hand, or wave goodbye, to pick up the phone (he never answered the phone anyway) … to say what he really wants to say when he wants to say it. We would appreciate any improvement and continue to hope and pray for full recovery.

~ ~ ~ ~ ~ ~ ~

One component of the above regimen that I never mentioned in my blog post was the daily coffee enema. It was a little too private for us to share at that time.

Coffee enemas have been found to have a positive effect on the gastrointestinal tract. They are said to reduce toxicity, clean the colon, increase energy levels and mood, help improve digestion, eliminate parasites, detoxify the liver, and are used at the Gerson Institute in the natural healing of cancer. There are said to be negative effects as well and one should consult a healthcare professional.

Anyway, though Mike hasn't had a coffee enema in a long time, we continue to this day with regular water enemas four to five times a week, just to keep things moving. When blogging about it or talking about it, I have always called it "our morning routine" or just "our routine."

I truly believe that the regular enemas for over two years have contributed to Mike's wellness, along with his very nutritious diet ... and of course, his positive attitude!

A Wonderful Gift Indeed—August 12, 2012

It was my birthday last week. I expected to receive some cards and gifts from family and friends and homemade cards, flowers, and a gluten-free birthday cake from my kids, like so many wonderful birthdays before. But, first thing in the morning, I prayed that I would receive something unexpected. As much as I love all that other stuff, I prayed for something more, something really big. I prayed that Mike would show some sign of improvement. He has been so diligent with his new diet and all the homeopathic remedies that I really wanted for my birthday a sign that Mike's efforts were paying off so he and the rest of us would be encouraged. That, to me, would be the ultimate birthday present.

I watched him closely all day. I waited to see something happen ... perhaps a few fingers would unfold, or maybe he would lift an arm or something. I listened closely to observe any improvements in his speech, but there weren't any. There weren't any changes at all. He seemed the same as he was the day before.

The next day as I pondered my birthday and the gift I wanted but didn't get, a light came on in my head as I realized that just spending the day with Mike was a gift. Every day I have with him is a splendid gift. And, what's more, Mike was the same as the day before ... he wasn't any worse. This, my gift, was a wonderful gift indeed!

Oswald Chambers says on my birthday (August 5): "What God calls us to cannot be definitely stated, because His call is simply to be His friend to accomplish His own purposes ... If we are in fellowship and oneness with God and recognize that He is taking us into His purposes, then we will no longer strive to find out what His purposes are. As we grow in the Christian life, it becomes simpler to us, because we are less inclined to say, 'I wonder why God allowed this or that?' And we begin to see that the compelling purpose of God lies behind everything in life, and that God is divinely shaping us into oneness with that purpose. A Christian is someone who trusts in the knowledge and the wisdom of God, not in his own abilities. If we have a purpose of our own, it destroys the simplicity and the calm, relaxed pace which should be characteristic of the children of God."

Grace Like Rain on a Really Hot Day—August 24, 2012

We were a little bit late for church last Saturday night. It was just a few minutes, but we were late and I didn't want to be late because Nathan was playing the drums and I didn't want to miss a minute of the music. Nevertheless, I felt rushed. I feel rushed a lot. It takes me and Mike a long time to do anything ... to get ready to go out, to get ready for bed, to get up and ready in the morning.

It took us a full hour to get ready to go get Madison from the airport earlier that day. Madison was in Edmonton for almost a week for the Canadian national ball hockey tournament and I was excited to go pick her up. Mike decided he wasn't going to come; he said he would lie down and have a little nap while I was gone. But first, he needed to go to the washroom. He also wanted to brush his teeth, have his face and hands washed, and blow his nose. Then I helped him to the couch to lie down. After about five minutes of arranging pillows here and there, he couldn't get comfortable, so I sat him back up and told him to come with me to the airport, and he could sleep on the way.

I put his socks and shoes on and we walked to the car. Believe it or not, that all took one hour, so now we were running late for the airport. I drove fast (faster than usual) and we got there on time, but had to wait about forty-five minutes for Madison's hockey stick to show up in the fragile-baggage claim. And this is what put us behind for church.

Earlier, while I fed Mike his lunch, he and I visited with Erin in the living room. Erin and I listened to fitness music and chose songs we liked for new playlists we both need for our fitness classes. We were having a wonderful, relaxing time, but had to wrap things up abruptly when I realized we needed to get ready to go to the airport.

Lunch was late that day, because Mike and I took Molly to the dike for a swim. Mike and I were taking care of the dog because Madison was away. We were in the middle of a heat wave and in order to keep the dog cool for a few hours and get her some exercise, we thought a swim was a good idea and that's what made our lunch late.

Molly had to wait though, because our nephew Luke had a

soccer game in the morning and we decided last minute to go (not really last minute—that would be out of the question— more like an hour before). Mike insisted to forgo his morning routine of drinks and Budwig Protocol to get to the game ... we still missed the first half. But that was okay, because the game ran late and that's why Molly had to wait.

It was a great day, but I'm not going to lie: a busy day like that is very exhausting for me and I can get frustrated. Plus, it was the hottest week of the year and that wasn't helping either. But regardless of the temperature, getting Mike here and there, in and out of the vehicle, to and from his wheelchair, up and down from the sofa, to the washroom, dressed and undressed, in and out of bed, from his left side to his right side, and so on and so forth can be a little wearing to say the least.

But that night at church when we sang "Hallelujah, grace like rain falls down on me. Hallelujah, all my stains are washed away ... they're washed away" (Chris Tomlin's rendition of "Amazing Grace"), it didn't matter that we were late. God's greatest gift to me—His grace ... His undeserved mercy and love—was all I needed to sing about, and I forgot about being late and the hurried feeling I felt five minutes before we got there. My energy was renewed, my attitude improved, and peace replaced the hurry.

In the words of another great song, the old hymn, "God's grace is greater than anything," including my rushed and hurried day, including a debilitating disease like ALS, including the imperfections of this world, including the trials of our lives. God's grace is greater than all these things, and it's really what I need the most to overcome the above and press on every day.

My, How Time Flies—September 3, 2012

Why does time have to fly? Why can't it crawl, or walk, or stroll … or even jog? Why does it have to fly? Time flies, so I guess it has wings, and what I've noticed as it gains momentum, it just goes faster and faster.

I remember when my children were little, mothers with older children would tell me to enjoy it while it lasts, because time flies and before you know it, they're all grown up. I would politely say something like, "Oh really?" But inside I was rolling my eyes and saying something like, "Whatever, lady." I take it back now and I wish I could turn the clock back a little too.

It feels just like yesterday I dropped my youngest child off at kindergarten. I cried then and I cried last week when we dropped her off at university. I will always be my children's mother and I hope they will always need me to some degree, but a chapter in my life has just come to an end and I'm a little sad.

Some parents are happy when their last one leaves the nest, but I'm just not ready for it yet. It's the end of child rearing I guess and that was my job, my joy, the biggest and best assignment of my life. In the twenty-three years that I have been a mom, I have made hundreds of peanut butter and jam sandwiches, I have driven to hundreds of practices, and I've given hundreds of pep talks. I've done thousands of loads of laundry; I have given thousands of good night kisses; and said thousands of late-night prayers. I have baked dozens of cookies and cupcakes, I have made dozens of Halloween costumes, I have thrown dozens of birthday parties, and I have bandaged dozens of scraped knees. Dance recitals and public speaking contests, hockey games and field trips, Christmas concerts and school plays, and on and on the list goes … most mothers know exactly what I'm talking about.

This weekend at Luke's soccer game, I got so excited when he scored a goal and received the MVP (most valuable player) award at the end of the game. I thought to myself that perhaps my *child rearing* days are over, but my *child cheering* days aren't. I was at the same soccer field my children played at most Labour Day weekends and here I was again with the same grand purpose in life: to cheer for a young person I love and his teammates, and to celebrate with them their accomplishments, and encourage them when they make mistakes (at soccer and in life). I just wanted to yell out to the parents all around me, "Enjoy it while it lasts, because time flies and before you know it, they're all grown up!" (I'd overlook a little eye rolling.)

Yesterday, Erin sent me a picture and a post on Facebook. It was a picture of her ballet slippers she found in the drawer of a dresser I recently gave her. She said, "I was emptying out your dresser drawer when I found these. I can't believe you kept them! I have so many memories of you driving me to ballet and always stopping for a cone. I guess some things never change, eh? Ha-ha. I love you, Mom!"

Home, Sweet Home—September 23, 2012

Yesterday, we cleared out the remainder of our things and handed over the keys of our dream house to complete strangers. The house Mike and I always said we would grow old in together now belongs to other people. But it's okay, because what I have learned is that home is where the love is, or like the *Vancouver*

Province newspaper put it on their front page on Friday, "Home is Where the Parents Are."

When I picked up the paper and read the front page, I told Mike it's exactly what I was going to tell Madison. And it's exactly how I felt for years after I moved out and got married and had children. When I went to my parents' house, it always felt like home. It wasn't necessarily the house they lived in; it was being wherever they were. A visit to their refrigerator and a little nap on their couch and some encouraging words from them and that was home.

Anyway, Mike and I moved out of our house and in with Elanna, Peter, Michaela, and Luke in the middle of July. We definitely procrastinated and should have left sooner, but didn't want to leave the home we loved ... we held on as long as we could (we also held on for dear life to the railing of those stairs going up and down every morning and night). Even though we contemplated keeping our house and renting it out, we put it up for sale in June. It sold at the end of July ... the day after we took it off the market. We knew it was for the best, but when the subjects were removed at the end of August, it was very bittersweet.

Madison was a little out of sorts a couple of weeks leading up to her move to university and it didn't take us long to figure out why. I was sure it had something to do with moving away from home and not having her home to come home to at Christmas and for summer break. Not only that, she had to give her dog and cats away as well.

Molly was commonly referred to as "Madison's dog" when she was being disobedient. "Madison, your dog is down the road. Madison, your dog is digging a hole in the front yard. Madison, your dog is eating the cat's food."

When Molly was being good, she was "our" dog. Well, I dropped our dog off at her new home last week. Our friends, the Hardies, welcomed Molly into their home with open arms.

Even though we have had to give up our house, our dog and cats, lots of things, and some hopes and dreams, I still feel like the luckiest girl in the world. We have incredible kids, a beautiful granddaughter, and amazing family and friends. ALS can't take that away from us. Plus, our permanent home is in heaven … we're just passing through this place.

To our children: Home is where your parents are … wherever we are is home and you are always welcome home!

To Elanna, Peter, Michaela, and Luke: Thanks for welcoming us into your home and making your home our home … we love it here. Thanks to Peter and his friend Keven for renovating the bathroom to make it wheelchair accessible.

To the Hardies: Thanks for loving our dog Molly and giving her a great home. We miss her a lot already, but we are so happy she has you!

To Helen our neighbour and friend Ken: Thanks for taking care of our cats until we could find homes for them.

One last thought: The most important things in life aren't "things" at all!

> *"Do not store up for yourselves treasures on earth, where moths and vermin destroy, and where thieves break in and steal. But store up for yourselves treasures in heaven, where moth and vermin do not destroy, and where thieves do not break in and steal. For where your treasure is, there your heart will also be."*
> **Matthew 6:19-21**

~ ~ ~ ~ ~ ~ ~

I will never forget when I saw that old house up for sale. I called Mike right away. I told him, "The house I have always loved is up for sale, can we go look?" It was actually too small for our family, but we bought it anyway and made do. Mike liked it, but I knew he only agreed we'd buy it because I loved it so much.

The process of selling it was really tough. Everything seemed to be slipping through our fingers. Emotionally, it was excruciating. The events leading up to the sale of our house had already almost crushed me and then this loss. We kept saying, "It's in God's hands." We had to leave everything there, we had no choice, but I held on too.

During this time, my friend Colleen kept calling and asking how we were doing. Colleen has a really good sense of timing. She listens well to that little voice in her, prompting her to call or send a message. When she calls me early in the morning and suggests we pray for my parents who are out on the mission field, I don't ask why she is calling so early or let her know she woke me up; I just agree.

During this particular time, Colleen kept saying, "Chris wants to do something for you. You've got to get him to do something for you. He wants to help." Chris and Colleen were our business partners for five years. We owned "Fitness Works," a fitness studio together. Colleen and Chris are a little older than us and very wise. Shortly after entering into a business arrangement with them (about twenty years ago), we learned they were even more capable, more competent, and smarter than we already knew them to be.

I'm not really great at accepting or asking for help (that darn pride), so I kept saying, "We're okay, we're okay." Although, I finally did tell Colleen if something came up, Chris would be the first to know ... sure enough, something came up.

When we got a decent offer for our lovely little abode, I admitted it was for the best and a weight was lifted. It was a lot of work to take care of Mike and a home and yard and a million other things. The potential buyers had a home inspector, a plumber, and an electrician take a look at the house ... everything went well and then they wanted the backyard scanned for an oil tank.

"Seriously? There's no way there's going to be an oil tank buried in the backyard ... That's ridiculous," I told Mike.

Sure enough, a huge oil tank was buried in the backyard. It was common for those old houses to still have oil tanks buried in the backyard ... we had no idea. So the whole yard had to be dug up and the oil tank removed (it filled the dump truck it was loaded into). Permits had to be purchased, the soil had to be tested for contamination by the fire department, and men had to be hired to do the job.

You know about the straw that broke the camel's back? Well, this was going to be that straw, but thankfully, Chris took care of it. Chris worked alongside our realtors, a father and son team Art and Nathan who had already gone above and beyond and were pillars of strength for us throughout the whole process. And good ol' Jim from next door who was always there to help, as well. Chris just stepped in and took over along with these men and got the job done. He supervised everything and came by every day for a week and took care of all the details. The soil was not contaminated and we all gave thanks in the end, and Mike and I still give thanks for these men!

Rocky Mountain High—October 5, 2012

The Golden Ears Mountains are what make our town of Maple Ridge so beautiful. I can't imagine this place without them.

When I used to drive my children to school when we lived on the other side of town, we turned off our street and headed north on Cottonwood toward Dewdney Trunk Road where we got a perfect view of the Golden Ears. I would tell my children, "Just look at those mountains!" and I would use words like "breathtaking, spectacular, amazing, gorgeous." My kids would say things like, "Yah, sure mom," or "Are you okay, mom?" I think they even told me to "gear down" a few times. But turning the corner and facing that beauty straight on really did take my breath away.

Today, I got a good long look at the Golden Ears. There is no snow on them right now, but it's only a matter of time. For ten months out of the year, there is snow on those mountains and after a fresh dusting, it's like, "Wow, did you get a look at those Ears this morning?" Without snow, they look naked ... all chiselled and really strong looking. It's like, "Where do you work out?"

I have only climbed the Ears once—with Mike, Peter, Colleen and Chris, and our niece Jenny from Toronto. (When any family members come to visit, Mike assumes they want to climb the mountain ... only some have taken him up on his challenge.)

Mike has climbed the Ears a bunch of times, including one time with our three kids and a couple of their friends.

It's a treacherous climb, but reaching the top gets you super high in more ways than one. You're on top of the world and it's incredibly invigorating, to say the least.

This past weekend, Mike and I and my mom and dad drove to Calgary to visit Madison at university and watch a couple of her hockey games. It's a really long drive—about twelve hours—but the views are spectacular. It's mountains and valleys all the way across BC and a little way into Alberta; the Rockies spit you out just before Calgary and then it starts getting flat.

I can become very emotionally charged when I am surrounded by mountains. They remind me how small I really am and how grand God is. They also make me think about the highs and lows of life ... the mountain-top experiences and the times spent in the deep valleys.

Our reading from *My Utmost for His Highest* in the morning on October 1, the day we drove home, says, "We have all experienced times of exaltation on the mountain, when we have seen things from God's perspective and have wanted to stay there. But God will never allow us to stay there …We are not made for the mountains, for sunrises, or for the other beautiful attractions in life—those are simply intended to be moments of inspiration. We are made for the valley and the ordinary things of life, and this is where we have to prove our stamina and strength."

I dedicate this blog post to our friends Neil and Donna. Neil had PLS for six years and was recently diagnosed with ALS. Our hearts go out to you, with love and prayers.

> *"I have told you these things, so that in Me you may have peace. In this world you will have trouble. But take heart! I have overcome the world."*
> **John 16:33**

Just One Word of Advice - October 19, 2012

While eating a piece of toast all smeared with honey and butter the other day, I was reminded of a childhood memory. When I visited my grandparents, I would climb up on their kitchen counter and help myself to their soda crackers and cover them with honey and eat them. Sometimes I would eat them right there while sitting on the counter and sometimes I would fill a plate and take them somewhere else to eat them and then go back for more when I was done. I love honey and I loved my grandparents, and on that grey, rainy day while sitting with Mike eating my toast, I got a little choked up and with one of those smiles you can't contain, I told him about my memories of soda crackers and honey on my grandma's kitchen counter.

This fond memory filled my heart with joy and brought a sense of thankfulness. Joy and thankfulness go hand in hand and I had to wonder if I was really experiencing those things very much lately. Sure, I thank the Lord every day for a big long list of things. I rattle that list off and quickly move on to my bigger list of requests; I have it down to a science.

Mike thanking God for ALS shortly after his diagnosis has stuck with me and has caused me to check my own attitude. Mike wasn't thankful for something he didn't want, like ALS, because he was going to lose the use of his arms and legs and because his speech was going to be greatly impaired and because swallowing was going to become a huge issue—of course not! What he went on to say was that he was thankful because ALS was going to cause him to rely more on God. Mike was wise and right; here we are a year and a half later and ALS has caused us to rely more on God.

When our son Nathan first started playing hockey, Mike and I would give him advice before every game. "Keep your head up." "Stay close to your man." "Pass the puck." "Encourage your team mates," and so on. Eventually, there was nothing we could say. He did all of those things and more, better than we could expect. So, this was the advice I started giving him, "Every time you step out on that ice, give thanks to the Lord." Then it just became, "Give thanks." After a while, all I had to say was; "Just one word of advice, Nathan," and he would say, "Yes, mom."

Later, I used the same "Just one word of advice" with Madison before every hockey game and I still do. An attitude of gratitude was something we taught our children because it would serve them well in life … in sports, in work, in relationships—in the good times and the really tough times.

The other day, shortly after I finished my delicious toast and after I finished reminiscing about my grandparents' place and the crackers and honey I ate on their kitchen counter, I checked Facebook and found a message from Madison. "My tape job this weekend." She attached a picture of the taped blade of her stick with the words "Give Thanks" written on it.

In This Together—October 28, 2012

Almost every day someone asks me how Mike is doing. When I'm at the gym or at the grocery store or at the bank, someone I know asks me about Mike. I usually stare at the person and smile, while I think about what I am going to say. It's such a hard question to answer, because physically Mike isn't that well, but in every other way, he is very well. Sometimes, I say he is great, sometimes good, sometimes okay … it's like, What do I say?

Mike can't really walk (he walks a little bit with his walker—really slow and shaky). He can't lift his arms or move his hands and fingers on his own. He is hard to understand … his speech is really impaired and he has swallowing issues as well. He can't scratch an itch or wipe his nose or feed himself or dress himself or shave or shower. Even so, Mike is still the most positive person I know. The only thing that frustrates him is not being able to verbally communicate the way he would like to. And yet, he laughs a lot at himself and at me. He'll say, "Scratch my eyebrow," and I'll say, "You want some pie now? Sorry, dear, we don't have any pie." He looks at me like what are you talking about, and then we laugh.

I feel honoured to be Mike's primary caregiver, but it's a lot of work. It's completely exhausting at times and backbreaking at times as well. It's tested my patience like nothing else. Sometimes I get frustrated but I try not to let it show. I try to be nice all the time, but find that a challenge once in a while.

Taking care of a grown man leaves little room for anything else; needless to say, my life has changed dramatically. It's just the way it is. I'm not mad or resentful or sad. If I think for a second how I'd like my life back, I shake my head and remind myself that Mike is the one with ALS. I always tell him, "We're in this together," but he is the one with the debilitating illness and has a good reason to be mad or resentful or sad ... but he is not. He is very content and I am humbled, again and again.

Shortly after Mike was diagnosed, our dear friend Pamela gave us a very wonderful gift—a donation of four hours of home care a week. We didn't need it right away and even when we could have used it, Mike wasn't ready. I finally told Mike that I was ready and in August, we started getting help once a week.

Voltaire is Mike's home care nurse and is at Mike's beck and call on Wednesdays from 10:00 a.m. till 2:00 p.m. He gives Mike his breakfast and a shave and a shower and brushes his teeth. Voltaire gives a perfect shave. He reclines Mike in his chair, lathers on the shave cream, and slowly removes every hair on his face, running back and forth to the sink in the washroom to rinse his razor.

Mike says Voltaire gives the best shave and I give him the best shower. Well, that's no surprise, when I give him a shower he calls it, "wet T-shirt time" (I usually end up as wet as him). He also really enjoys the long head massage I give him when

I shampoo his hair. I scrub him from head to toe and when I'm done, he always says the same thing, "I feel like a million bucks!"

Pat came out for a couple of weeks in September (right after Aileen was here to help us move Madison). Pat's timing was perfect; she took care of Mike every day while I packed up our house in preparation for our move.

I would get Mike ready in the morning and then take him to her motel, where she spoiled him with the meals and snacks he really likes, and gave him back massages. They did crossword puzzles and went for walks and watched whatever Mike wanted to watch on TV. After a long day of packing, I would go home and change and then Elanna and I would walk up to the motel and pick Mike up and walk him home.

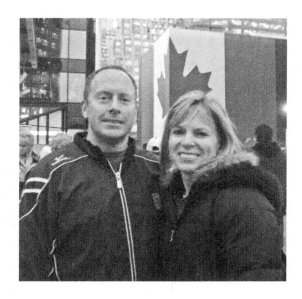

Mike and Nadine in Vancouver, Winter Olympics 2010

Elanna also helps us out at home. She offers to give Mike his breakfast or dinner sometimes, so I can have a shower or make something to eat for myself. She folds our laundry and does our dishes sometimes as well.

I recently thought to myself, with the help of three women plus Voltaire, Mike is well cared for; but it's come to that time for more regular home care support (probably a little overdue). The community nurse and occupational therapists have been in a few times to prepare for more home care support starting soon. I must say, this is one of the hardest things we have had to do so far.

I want to be there for Mike all the time, but I know it's important for both of us to get more help. It's another adjustment we have to make and trying to keep in line with Mike's positive attitude, I'm sure we will be fine.

Rescued—November 9, 2012

When Erin was in grade six, she was diagnosed with Legg-Calvé-Perthes disease. Legg Perthes is a condition where the supply of blood to the hip joint is interrupted, causing the hip joint to collapse to some degree because of bone mass loss in the femoral head. It affects about one in twelve hundred children who are typically very active and athletic, and only one in four are girls.

Erin was in full leg casts and then leg braces until the end of grade seven. During that time, she had a couple of surgeries and was in a lot of pain. I remember how helpless I felt as her mother. I was "failing" as her mom, because I couldn't stop the pain or prevent her from going through what she was going through.

Shortly after one of Erin's surgeries, I received a card in the mail from my cousin Kim who wrote, "'So do not fear for I am with you; do not be dismayed for I am your God. I will strengthen you and help you; I will uphold you with My righteous right hand.' Isaiah 41:10."

I was already hanging on to this verse for dear life, but getting the card in the mail with these words was confirmation that God wanted me to know that He meant what He said and He would help me and was indeed already helping me … and He would give me the strength to help Erin through a very tough time.

Many times since then I have called out to the Lord for help for different reasons. Since Mike was diagnosed with ALS, I have called out for help a lot, sometimes in desperation, and God has never failed to help. Sometimes His help is subtle and sometimes it is not subtle; regardless, I am always amazed at His creative ways of rescuing me in His perfect timing. And I am ever so thankful that He is always with me and that He gives me strength every day.

Erin still suffers from the effects of Legg Perthes, but has overcome so much. She will have to have hip replacement surgery soon, but continues to persevere and does what she can. She has been teaching fitness classes since she was sixteen years old and recently graduated with her Education Degree and is now a French Immersion schoolteacher working in the schools in our community.

Chapter 11
Golden

A Couple of Chickens and a Shower Chair— November 20, 2012

I don't like clutter; I don't like a big mess. I like space and things in their place. We have always lived in relatively small homes and Mike learned early on that I don't like clutter. When we lived in our first one-room apartment, Mike told me a story about a guy who went to the town advisor for advice. He told the wise advisor, "My house is too small. What should I do?"

The town advisor told him to go home and bring one of his chickens in the house and come back in a week. After a week, the guy went back and said, "My house isn't any bigger and the chicken is pooping all over the place and stinking up the joint."

The town advisor told him to go home and bring another chicken into his house and come back again in another week. The guy did what he was told and came back after a week. He said, "My house isn't any bigger and it's a mess!"

The advisor sent him home and told him to bring in a pig as well; then it was another pig and then a goat and then another goat and then a cow and so on. When the guy went back he said, "Look Buddy, my house isn't any bigger and these animals are getting on my last nerve!" The advisor told him to go home and let all the animals out of his house.

When the guy went back to the wise guy a week later, he said, "Wow, I didn't realize my house was so big!"

Over the years, anytime I mentioned any little thing about our small house, Mike would say, "Have I ever told you the story about the guy whose house was too small?"

I would say, "Yes!" and then he would say, "You haven't heard this one." And he would tell the story, but use different animals or put them in a different order or give the guy a different name, etc.

On Saturday, Mike and I went to Nathan's soccer game. We took Leah with us so Nathan could go early to warm up with his team … that's what we usually do. It was pouring rain and we were thankful that the field had some shelter, but it was a little way away from the parking lot, so we were pretty wet when we got there.

Like many soccer games we have attended over the years, we were wet and cold. We huddled under the shelter with the other fans and watched an exciting first half. Nathan was playing great and Mike wasn't about to take his eyes off the game until half time, when he looked at me with a look of urgency and told me he had to go pee.

I grabbed our things and we ran. The washrooms weren't that far away, but our car was closer and I keep a jar under the seat for emergencies. Unfortunately, we didn't quite make it. I felt sick to my stomach and so defeated.

My husband is a smart man. He is wise and witty and competent. He was a good athlete and a hard worker. He raised three great kids and is well respected in our community. Here he sat in his wheelchair unable to get to the bathroom on time, a very low moment in a man's life, for sure. Thank the Lord it was pouring rain and we were all soaking wet anyway.

Leah knew something was up, but we kept telling her everything was fine. I helped her in to the van and buckled her up. Then I helped Mike out of his wheelchair and to his seat, beside Leah (behind the driver's seat where he always sits). We struggled more than usual to get Mike in his seat. At one point, his leg gave out on him and he just dropped. I grabbed him with both my arms around him and with all my might I tried to lift him back up to standing. With the help of a couple of men who saw us struggling, we got Mike in his seat and we left.

If Leah hadn't been with us, I know I would have lost it. With tears rolling down my cheeks, I kept a smile on my face and kept reassuring Leah that Granddad was just fine (she couldn't see my tears). I was amazed at Mike's ability to stay calm and keep his head up. He seemed just fine like I kept telling Leah.

When we got home, Leah went upstairs to visit her cousins Michaela and Luke, and Mike and I went into our new little basement suite and closed the door so we could get cleaned up. Our small space has recently gotten smaller and has started to resemble a medical supply store.

We have two wheelchairs (one from the ALS Society that we have been using for a long time, but isn't the right size, and a new-to-us used top-of-the-line wheelchair our friend Denise has lent us). We have two shower chairs (one the occupational therapist brought us a while ago and a nice new one on wheels that Pat got us). We also have Mike's walker and stationary bike in the room, as well as our table on wheels and all our normal household stuff. Anyway, it's been a little crowded lately, to say the least.

While we were getting cleaned up, I couldn't stop crying … I was so upset about what had happened. Mike who was fully composed and who hates to see me cry, looks around the room and then looks at me and, as clear as day, says, "And then the town wise guy said, 'Bring in another shower chair.'"

All You Need Is Love—December 4, 2012

This is my one-hundredth blog post and I dedicate it to our family and friends. The support, the encouragement, the prayers, the concern, the comforting words, the food, the money, the gifts, the help, the fundraisers, and so on; it's all summed up in one word: LOVE. We thank you from the bottom of our hearts!

Something I have learned about myself over the last little while is that I can be quite selfish. Taking care of Mike full time has revealed selfishness in me I wouldn't have realized otherwise. I delight in caring for Mike; he is my husband and I love him very much. But here is my question to myself, Do I love me more? Ultimately, my needs are quite often first and foremost on my mind, to be quite honest.

For a while, I had no problem giving up a lot of things in order to take the best care of my beloved. But when the novelty of that wore off and my inner child started throwing a temper tantrum because she wasn't getting what she wanted, I had to give my inner child a "time out" and ponder what love was really about.

Jesus says something about love that strikes a chord in me. In John 15:13, He says, "Greater love has no one than this, that he lay down his life for his friends." Jesus knew what He was talking about because He knew His future and the very reason He came to earth—to suffer the cruelest death on a cross for His friends … the greatest example of love. But in this verse, Jesus wasn't just talking about the great love He had for his friends (and all of mankind); He was telling all mankind how they must love one another as well. In the verse right before it,

He says, "My command is this: Love each other as I have loved you."

When I was a child, I didn't need to hear the words "I love you" to know that I was loved. The actions of those caring for me, my parents and grandparents and aunts and uncles, were enough for me to know I was loved. I also found out quickly that I didn't have to do anything to earn their love. They just loved me for who I was because I belonged to them. They put aside their needs for mine and rearranged their lives to suit me … and that's what most parents and grandparents and aunts and uncles do.

At the age of eighteen, our son Nathan announced that he was going to be a dad. After his big announcement, he showed us how "big" he was by laying down his life for his new baby. He quit the high-level hockey team he was on. He shelved any plans of going to college and/or travelling. He started getting up at the crack of dawn to go to a job he didn't like in order to raise a beautiful baby girl. His daughter Leah knows she is well loved, because his life revolves around her and she means everything to him.

Love is an action word. It means putting someone else before self; it's about giving something up for another person and not expecting anything in return.

When Mike first started needing help walking and going up the stairs and getting dressed and eating, etc., we gained a new appreciation for caregivers. We would quite often say, "God bless the April Cartwrights of the world!" April Cartwright is a woman Mike went to elementary school with and is now a friend of both of ours on Facebook. As a single parent, she has had to give up everything for her daughter with autism.

Her daughter, now in her twenties, needs constant care and attention and always will.

Our friends, Michelle and Dave also have a daughter with special needs. Watching them with their daughter is a lesson in love. They are so patient and kind and I'm sure their daughter knows she is loved beyond measure and it's inspiring to say the least.

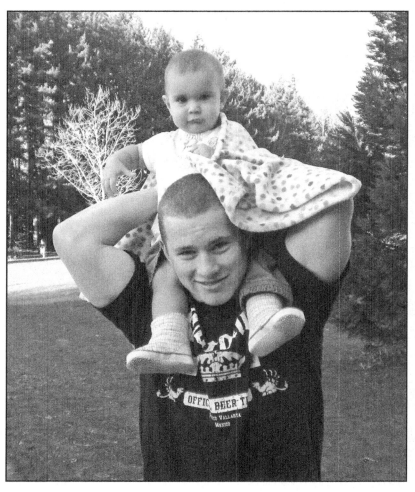

Nathan and Leah

My dad just returned from Malawi again where he, in his mid-seventies, still goes to feed orphans and drill wells. He and my mom have laid down their lives for their "friends." Just like other people who have chosen to care for someone else's child. Or like those caring for their own children, or an aging parent, or a sick friend. Or like the parents, sisters and brothers, children, nieces, nephews, aunts, uncles, cousins, friends, and me who care for a guy named Mike with ALS.

"If I have the gift of prophecy and can fathom all mysteries and all knowledge, and if I have a faith that can move mountains, but have not love, I am nothing."
I Corinthians 13:2

Communication Breakdown—December 16, 2012— by Mike Sands

Language has been around for almost as long as man has existed. There are close to seven thousand languages worldwide. With the large number of languages in existence coupled with the different dialects, it stands to reason that problems will arise when communicating between people.

An example of this occurred in the Sudan a few years ago. An advertiser posted on a billboard three pictures side by side. The first picture showed a bunch of dirty clothes. The middle picture had a box of Tide detergent, and the last picture showed the same clothes but now they were clean after using the Tide. The problem was that in Sudan, the Sudanese people read from right to left, not left to right as we do in Canada. This "miscommunication" was an obvious embarrassment to the advertisers.

Another example of where language was "miscommunicated" occurred in Russia during the 1800s when Czarina Maria Feodorovna once saved the life of a man by transposing a single comma in a warrant signed by her husband, Alexander III. The warrant exiled a criminal to imprisonment and death in Siberia. On the bottom of the warrant, the czar had written: "Pardon impossible, to be sent to Siberia." Maria Feodorovna changed the punctuation so that her husband's instructions read: "Pardon, impossible to be sent to Siberia." By altering the document, the Czarina caused a "miscommunication" between the czar and the jailer. The criminal was set free.

Closer to home in North America, there was a comedy duo of George Burns and Gracie Allen that ran their act from the early days of vaudeville in the 1920s until Gracie's death in 1964. Burns and Allen, as they were known, built their act on miscommunication—largely on the part of the ditzy Gracie, who always misinterpreted anything straight man George said. An example of miscommunication between the two occurred one time when George came home and noticed Gracie putting a bunch of flowers in a vase. George asked Gracie where she got the flowers. Gracie replied: "I went to visit Edna Rigby in the hospital, and you told me if I was to visit her in the hospital, then I should take her flowers. So I took them."

I just arrived back from the European country of Bulgaria where I received stem cell treatment for my ALS. The treatment is not offered in Canada, as it is deemed controversial. The procedure involved taking healthy stem cells from one section of my body (the bone at the top of my right butt cheek) and transferring the cells to an unhealthy section (my neck). I was transferred from a gurney to an operating table. I was placed on my side so they could drill my butt cheek.

ALS has caused severe muscle loss in my arms, and therefore, lying on my side causes me great pain unless I place a pillow between my arms and my side. Being in the foreign country of Bulgaria made any conversation ripe for misinterpretation, plus my slurred speaking didn't help either. Some of the medical staff attending me barely spoke English, so I was hard pressed to figure out how I was going to communicate to them that I needed a pillow under my arm.

I said out loud to anyone who would listen, "I need a pillow," while pointing to under my arm.

The nurse replied, "No pills while surgery."

I thought to myself, "What?" I asked for a pillow and he thinks I want a pill. I then saw a stack of hospital pyjamas about five metres away on a shelf. I said out loud, "I need those pyjamas," while pointing to my underarm.

He replied, "Momma not allowed in surgery."

I said I wanted pyjamas and he thought I said I want my momma.

All of a sudden, I could relate to women in labour who become very annoyed with the medical staff ... I've heard women say they feel like they could punch someone in the face (including their husband).

But that was not how I was going to deal with this situation.

I thought, "What would Jesus do?" Yes, now I remember; Matthew 5:29, and Jesus sayeth; "Turn the other cheek." So I used all my strength and turned my hips lifting my left butt cheek so that it was flapping in the breeze for all to see.

Yes, Jesus would be proud; I had turned the other (butt) cheek.

Go, Fight, Win!—December 29, 2012

We had a really nice Christmas. A popular song claims that Christmas is the most wonderful time of the year, but for some it's not. It can be a very sad and lonely time of the year for many people, and my heart goes out to those who don't experience comfort and joy at Christmas.

Some people are away from the ones they dearly love, so it makes me appreciate every Christmas spent with family. I savour the moments and wish time would stand still for just a little while.

Our children are grown up, but it's still so much fun to watch them open presents and it's neat that they are more excited about what they give than what they get. They appreciate the good food, especially the turkey and gravy, and they enjoy spending time with each other and the rest of the family. There is usually lots of laughter, lots of sweet treats, stories, games, and someone snoozing on the couch or in the middle of the living room floor. Having a three-year-old granddaughter around as well makes Christmas extra special and we just couldn't ask for anything more.

It's these special times together that can give someone with an illness the desire and determination to fight for his life and live to experience it all over again next year … and the next year and the one after that. How do I know? I know because I am watching a very courageous man do exactly that.

To go all the way to Bulgaria to receive a medical treatment that is still fairly new and may or may not produce positive results is courageous. Our motto is, "We will do whatever we can and let God do the rest … and may His will be done!" We are all very hopeful, but before we left for Bulgaria, Mike said, if nothing else, it will be a wonderful pre-Christmas vacation to a beautiful destination.

We feel so blessed to have been able to travel across the globe to be treated by some of the very best doctors in the world. We couldn't have done it without the help of Elanna who came with us, and without the help of my parents who initiated the trip and took care of all the travel arrangements (with the help of their friends who have the connections with the doctors in Bulgaria and are helping many people, including those with MS and ALS find medical relief through their society, The Reformed Multiple Sclerosis Society). We are also so thankful for the prayers and support of all our family and friends and to Erin's friend Jamie for hosting a fundraiser for us to help with some expenses.

Over the Christmas holidays, Audrey and Gregg arranged two friendly hockey games for their kids and friends. Everyone paid ten bucks (a bargain) to play the game of scrimmage. Audrey and Gregg passed on all the proceeds to Project Wellness, which was an added bonus.

The games were great entertainment for those of us watching, but what I noticed right away was the competitiveness of all the players, especially our two, Nathan and Madison. It was a friendly game against good friends they have known all their lives, but when the puck dropped, the game was ON! It got me thinking, it's in the genes … our three children are just like their dad: very competitive. Mike is very competitive in sports and other things in life, including illness. It's like, "Go, Fight, Win!" almost all the time. Their attitude is, "I will not be beat!"

The doctors say it can take one to two months to observe any results from the stem cell treatment, so we will wait and see what happens. But regardless of what happens, we will not lose hope. With the advancements in medicine and the brilliant doctors out there and considering that all things are possible with God, we won't lose hope! And with the competitive spirit that Mike has, he won't stop fighting.

> *"Now all glory to God, who is able, through His mighty power at work within us, to accomplish infinitely more than we might ask or think."*
> **Ephesians 3:20, NLT**

A Good Hair Day—January 13, 2013

Well, it's a new year. Happy New Year! I like the New Year; it's like a fresh start. It's a time to reflect on the past, and anticipate the future; perhaps, set a few goals. For some, it's a time to make major changes and for others, it's a time to make a few minor adjustments. Not everyone makes New Year's resolutions, but many do. As a fitness instructor, I can vouch for the many who do … classes are overcrowded at the gym and the parking lot is packed.

I have made a few resolutions this year along with the one resolution I make every year, which is to eat less/pray more. I guess making the same resolution every year is an indication that I haven't had the greatest success, so I keep trying, just like the January gym goers who believe this year they will accomplish their fitness goals and exercise the other eleven months as well. I say, "Good for you! You can do it!"

As I pondered my list of resolutions this week, I decided to tweak my resolution of "eat less, pray more" to "eat less" (that stays) and "PRAISE more." I have been contemplating the past year and there is absolutely no way we could have made it through without the help of the Lord. We experienced more changes and more challenges last year than all the other years combined, and I know I would have snapped without Him. So many times, I called out to Him and He was there. So many times I couldn't call out, I had no voice, I had nothing, and He was there. I was convinced a long time ago that my Heavenly Father is always there, but it just seemed to be the theme of 2012. While remembering all the wonders He has done, I decided He deserves more praise.

One of my favourite Bible verses illustrates so well how God cares and how He knows His children and how much He values them: Matthew 10:29-31 says; "Are not two sparrows sold for a penny? Yet not one of them will fall to the ground outside your Father's care. And even the very hairs of your head are all numbered. So don't be afraid; you are worth more than many sparrows."

Speaking of hair, I will share a story of how one day I received a gift certificate from five dear friends to go get my hair done. It was very generous; it was enough for colour and a cut at the salon where I normally go for just a cut.

I booked my appointment in advance and when the day came, I was very excited to spend some time at the salon. Knowing that the cost was covered, I relaxed and enjoyed my makeover even more than usual. Three hours later, when I was all done and felt like a million bucks, I went to present my gift certificate to the receptionist. The receptionist told me that while I was having my hair done a woman called and told her that she saw me through the window in the salon chair while driving by; she'd been running some errands at the same strip mall. The receptionist said that my friend, I'll call her SB, gave her a credit card number and said she wanted to pay for my salon service that day. The receptionist told her I had a gift certificate, so SB said to charge her with any costs not covered by the gift certificate.

I didn't understand at first what the receptionist was telling me. After she explained it again, I couldn't believe it! I actually had to laugh ... I cried a little too. The gift certificate covered the bill plus tax, so the receptionist charged SB with the tip.

I don't believe this was a coincidence; I believe it was a set up. The Lord set me up again to deliver a profound message. He doesn't really care about my hair colour, but He does know every strand on my head, and He cares for me beyond measure. It wasn't about the money, because I had the money. It was another example of many this past year that proved how He is always with us and how He will always take care of us.

Jersey Day—January 20, 2013

Well, the boys are back on the ice ... it's like an answer to a prayer. Yesterday, Mike watched his team the Toronto Maple Leafs beat the Montreal Canadiens, and then he watched his other team the Vancouver Canucks get beat by the Anaheim Mighty Ducks. Our boy, Cory Schneider, didn't get off to the greatest start in net, but we're happy to have him for another season, and we'll be cheering for him again next game.

As the players have been on strike, it's been a long winter without the "Good ol' Hockey Game," but our motto is "better late than never" and, like Mike keeps telling us, he is bored. So in the morning, he put on his new Leafs T-shirt and sat in front of the set and waited for the puck to drop. Mike wasn't the only one waiting for the game to get going; it's like the people have been resuscitated. Everyone is smiling again and sporting their favourite hockey jersey.

Friday was jersey day at Erin Langton Elementary School, where Erin teaches grade seven French Immersion. It's also the school she and her brother and sister attended. It was jersey day at Laity View School where Luke and Michaela go. I thought it was a coincidence, but Erin told me it was jersey day at all the schools in the district.

I brought Erin her favourite jersey and gave her a lift to school in the morning. She was so excited that I was able to locate her old Colorado Avalanche jersey that she wore when she was a kid ... probably a thousand times. Erin is very small, so the jersey she got in grade four still fits her, with the exception of the sleeves, but she can wear it ... and she wore it on jersey day with great pride, just like she wore it in grades four through seven and beyond.

We were all big fans of the Colorado Avalanche when Joe Sakic was team captain. Erin started it; she was a huge fan and then she became Sakic's number one fan when he called her the day after she'd had hip surgery. Not only did he call her to wish her well, he sent her a signed jersey for Christmas. Erin's teacher, Mme. Dudley had some connections through a family member and arranged everything. Needless to say, we all became fans the day he called and we will never forget it. (We are also fans of Mme. Dudley who taught all three kids.)

Anyway, the signed Sakic jersey has never been worn and is in a safe place, and the little one Erin took to school the other day is well worn and has a story of its own. With enthusiasm, Erin reminded me about the day she got her treasured Colorado jersey. Erin, the gifted public speaker that she is, had competed that morning in the school's public speaking contest. She and her brother were big competitors with lots of ribbons to show for it. This particular speech was about the National Hockey League and Erin delivered it flawlessly. Mike and I of course were there to cheer her on and, without my knowledge, Mike later went and purchased the Colorado jersey for Erin and took it to her in the afternoon when he picked the kids up from school.

She continued to tell me how it was such a great surprise and how she thought she would never have a Colorado jersey because jerseys were so expensive. She said it was one of the best gifts she has ever received and it was from her favourite guy—her dad!

Erin has two valuable Colorado Avalanche jerseys; one is priceless and so are the memories!

P.S. For Nathan, it was a Boston Bruins jersey and his was signed by another one of our favourite players, Bobby Orr. Madison wore an Avalanche jersey like her sister. And they all had Vancouver Canucks jerseys of course.

Golden Boy—January 31, 2013

I think it's pretty cool that, with my blogger account, I can check to see how many people are reading and where they are from. For instance, I know there are seventeen people reading my blog right now. I can also see where they are from and what blog posts are being read. I can check what the numbers are for the day, week, month, and all time. I'm amazed at how people from all over the world are reading. Canada, USA, Sweden, Russia, UK, Germany, France, Ukraine, Australia, and Brazil are the top ten, to name just a few. People are reading from countries I haven't even heard of ... that's the magic of the internet! *ALS With Courage* is approaching fifty thousand hits, most of the hits from people I don't know. But here is what I do know; we are all in the same boat.

We are all in the same boat! There are no exceptions. We all experience trials of many kinds. That's life! But, you know what's been said about life? It's 10 percent what happens to us and 90 percent how we react. We have a choice how we live and how we react to the trials and the struggles and the difficulties of life ... it's a lot to do with attitude.

Mike continues to possess the most amazing attitude, along with his strong faith and incredible courage; he has something very special. To date, there's not been one "woe is me." He still tells jokes even though he has to spell them out (literally), because we don't understand. The laughs are delayed, but nevertheless, we laugh. He takes everything in stride and never complains. He is the same guy on the inside, perhaps an even better version of himself. He has allowed the fires to refine him into a beautiful masterpiece, and I just don't know how to express how incredible it is to watch. I feel so small and insignificant next to my "golden boy." It's humbling and I'm in awe.

"These trials will show that your faith is genuine. It is being tested as fire tests and purifies gold—though your faith is far more precious than mere gold. So when your faith remains strong through many trials, it will bring you much praise and glory and honour ..."
I Peter 1:7, NLT

Mike never focuses on what he can't do or what he has lost. He stays focused on what he can do and what he still has. On Sundays at 11:00 a.m., we sometimes watch Pastor Joel Osteen on TV, who said a couple of weeks ago, "As long as you have breath, you have purpose." Mike's purpose may have changed, and perhaps is even more significant now. He has become a great teacher and I, a student, still have a lot to learn.

P.S. Mike hasn't experienced any changes in his condition since the stem cell treatment he had on December 5, but we aren't discouraged about it: we are content and still hopeful. Whatever happens, God is with us and He is worthy of all our praise!

General Hospital—February 17, 2013—by Mike Sands

Hospitals have been around for a long time. Up until the beginning of the twentieth century, most hospitals were run through religious organizations. It was at this time in history that the public realized that government-run hospitals were necessary to ensure a more egalitarian, structured medical system. Formal hospitals were set up with access guaranteed to the public—provided the client was willing to pay. In Canada in the early 1960s, we moved to a publicly funded system as we realized healthcare was a necessity for all, not just for a privileged few, unlike in the United States where it's still pay as you go, or as Groucho Marx said, "In the US, a hospital bed is a parked taxi with the meter running."

As a Registered Nurse, I've been associated with the hospital setting for many years. I worked at Riverview Hospital for twelve years. Riverview was a hospital for the mentally ill. Mentally ill people often find themselves on the outer parameters of society, as they often do not fit in or conform to society's mores. I found this job to be very rewarding and very interesting. I particularly found it enjoyable and refreshing how many of them would speak their mind; they would say things that many of us thought but were afraid to say.

I remember hearing one story of a nurse coming into a patient's room to give him his antipsychotic injection. As the nurse walked in the room, the patient yelled at the nurse, "They treat us like dogs around here." The nurse yelled back, "That's nonsense. Now, rollover!"

The only problem I had working in a hospital was that whenever I wanted to call in sick, the boss would say, "Oh, you're sick? Why don't you come into work and we'll take a look at it."

With the onset of my ALS, I knew my days of serving patients were now going to be reversed. My second taste of hospitalization came last week when I was admitted to get a feeding tube put in. With ALS, the muscles in your throat become weakened. Swallowing becomes difficult and the need to supplement your nutrition becomes necessary.

The surgery only lasted fifteen minutes. I was then wheeled back to my room. With my dire diagnosis of ALS, the doctors are more liberal at doling out the pain medication. So I pretty much had free-reign with the morphine. The adage "too much of a good thing is not good" fits this situation.

Although I was pain free and as giddy as a schoolboy, morphine decreases your respirations. It makes you feel like there's an elephant on your chest ... it was terrible. Never again will I be tempted by the allure of morphine.

The guy in the next bed was on the same "morphine trip" I was on. As his wife sat by his bedside, his eyes fluttered open and he said to her, "You're beautiful." Flattered, she continued her vigil as he fell back to sleep. Later, he woke up and said to her, "You're cute." Startled she said, "What happened to 'beautiful'?" He said, "The morphine is starting to wear off."

My last night in the hospital, I was transferred to a room with three patients who all seemed to suffer with mental illness. I looked across the room at a man tied at the waist to the bed. He was struggling feverishly, to no avail, to get out of his bed. I thought of the irony between the two of us—me, unable to move a muscle and in control of all my mental faculties, and him, strong as an ox and not in his right mind.

Oh, what a team we could have made with his brawn and my brains ... we could've been a contender.

Don't Judge a Man by His ALS—February 20, 2013 — by Erin Sands

I'll never forget my first day of university ... ahh, sweet freedom! I felt so independent living on my own at the University of Fraser Valley dorms in Abbotsford. A brand new adventure and I was out in the real world.

On my first night away from home, I decided to go for a run

to scope out my new digs. I didn't know the area at all, so I just started running, not knowing where I was going or where I would end up. Fortunately, I came across a track. I was so excited, because I absolutely love running at the track. The stadium lights shone brightly and I was thrilled at my discovery. The only problem was there was this big fence that gave no access to the prime running real estate!

I figured they wanted to keep out all of the thugs and hoodlums who were up to no good. But I was just a sweet, innocent girl wanting to go for a run, so I decided I would hop the fence. As I began to scale this thing, I noticed that there was barbed wire at the top. I thought to myself "They must really want to keep these bad kids out." All of a sudden, two cops with big flashlights came running out at me. They yelled, "WHAT ARE YOU TRYING TO DO, YOUNG LADY?"

I told them with desperation in my voice "I just want to run on your track!" They looked at each other puzzled, and the officer then said, "This is not a track …. This is the Matsqui prison!"

I've come to learn to never judge a book by its cover, or a track by its bright lights. The same can be said for my dad. Most people talk to him like he is either deaf or a three-month-old baby. Even people he knows well will come over and yell very slowly "HELLLOOO MIKE, DO YOU REMEMBER ME?" Oh great, now they think he has amnesia too!

ALS rarely affects the brain. My dad may not be able to move his body, down a quarter chicken with fries at Swiss Chalet, or sing the lyrics to "I wear my sunglasses at night," but he is still the same big kid who taught my brother and me how to play Nicky-Nicky-Nine-Doors, the brainiac who helped me with all my homework, and the wise man who always has perfect advice. He's still the guy who encourages me when I am down and makes my stomach hurt from laughing at his hilarious jokes.

Today is my twenty-fourth birthday and I am so thankful for every single year and moment I have had to spend with this amazing man. From the first day I was born, he has loved and taken care of me, and ALS has never come in the way of that. He may be different physically, but he will always be the same old daddy!

So, two words of advice—Don't ever judge someone by their appearance AND if there is a huge fence with barbed wire, it's probably not a good idea to try hopping over it. You may just be breaking into a prison.

Most Valuable Dad—February 24, 2013 — by Madison Sands

When I was little, I wasn't the typical "let's play Barbies and then have a tea party" kind of girl. I had short messy hair, rode a two-wheeler up and down the street, and was often mistaken for "a cute little boy!"

Our mom and dad always had us kids in all kinds of sports … track, cross-country, soccer, ball hockey, rugby, etc.

When I was three, my mom registered me in a summer dance class, but that only lasted about two weeks … she realized the only reason I went was because McDonalds was right beside the dance studio.

A few years later, my parents put me in speed skating, but after refusing to wear those stupid tights, I wasn't allowed to compete, so that didn't last long.

It wasn't until I was eight years old when my dad came home and told me he finally signed me up for ice hockey.

My dad has always been a big part of my hockey career, and he is the main reason I got to where I am today. He would specifically work the night shift so he wouldn't miss a game. He was my number one critic, and if I sucked, oh, I'd hear about it. Even though he wasn't on the bench coaching, his opinion was most important to me. He was always hard on me, but I knew that it was only to help me get better. For example, when my dad picked me up from elementary school, he'd make me run laps at the high school track while waiting for my siblings to be dismissed. Or days when I was sick and had a game, he would hand me any kind of medicine and say, "Take this and let's go!" as I'd be throwing up in a bag on the drive there.

Most parents brag about their kids' report cards or honour roll list. Instead, my dad would pull out my stats and show them my point total. He'd show up to my class and tell the teacher I had an "appointment" and take me to the rink for "stick and puck" to prepare me for the big game I had that night. And every year at the parent-teacher interview when the teacher was explaining to him the things I needed to work on, his response was, "Yah, but have you seen her slap shot?"

At tournaments, he was the first to jump on the hotel bed, start a towel fight in the pool, and everyone knew when Mike Sands was picking MVP for the opposing team. It wasn't the star of the game who got it, but the one who tried the hardest.

He is not your typical dad; he is more like a friend. From day one, he was always there. He taught me how to hold a stick, tie my skates, and even throw a punch. And his motto, which I am sure my brother, sister, and I will pass on to our children, was

"If you aren't practising, someone else is, and when they meet you, they will beat you!"

This past September I left home for university to play the sport I love. It was very difficult, because I left behind the man that I love suffering with something I'm not able to help him with … and he was always there to help me. But reminiscing helped me realize that it's what he always loved watching me do, and what he was preparing me to do for all these years.

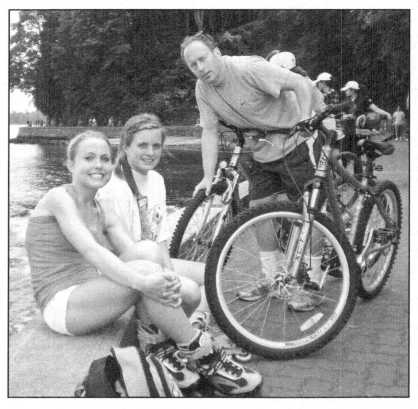

Mike with Erin and Madison at the Seawall in Vancouver

Chapter 12
A Dog's Love

I've been struck by lightning a few times ... NOT really. But I feel like I have. Not like the electrocution part of being struck by lightning but like the outward glow of a quick jolt of a bolt; perhaps it might also be thought of as an "aha moment."

I've never used the term "aha moment" until now, but it's the best way to describe those profound, cognitive occurrences. Right on the spot, just like that, your mind is opened up, and wisdom and understanding pour in.

I remember one major jolt of a bolt like it was yesterday, but it was a long time ago: September 12, 2001. The only reason I know the date is because it was the day after 9/11. I accompanied a friend downtown to an appointment that day. While she was in her two-hour appointment, I went for a walk. Robson Street wasn't the usual busy hub of Vancouver ... it was understandably quiet. It was a nice sunny day, but a sombre one for sure.

There weren't many cars on the road, but when I stepped off the curb to cross the street, I was struck ... by lightning ... that is.

It feels like I stood there for quite some time as I processed the aha moment, but I think I kept walking. I see myself with a glow around me like angels were accompanying me, and maybe they were, but the Spirit definitely was speaking to my soul.

Directly in front of me, sitting on the sidewalk, was a young man and a dog. They had a sign that said something about needing money and food. While I have never had anything against people asking for money and I've never had anything against dogs, I have had something against people with dogs asking for money. My closed mind always thought things like, "Let the dog go; he can probably do better on his own." Or, "How can you take care of a dog, when you can't take care of yourself?"

Anyway, those thoughts changed that day when my mind

was opened and wisdom and understanding were poured in. Aha! I knew at that moment it was all about love. I walked straight up to the guy and said hello.

I've never had a problem talking to someone on the street asking for money ... I don't like to refer to them as "beggars," because most just ask, not beg. I think "asker" is more appropriate. Mike and I would always take granola bars downtown with us when we went, because we didn't like ignoring the askers. Mike also made sure to put change in his pocket and he used to get those McDonald bucks and give those out too. Years ago, one Christmas Eve when I was very pregnant, Mike and Elanna took a hundred of those paper bucks (that don't exist anymore) downtown and gave them out. Elanna still talks about that Christmas Eve as being one of her most memorable.

Anyway, the asker I encountered on September 12 was a well-spoken, fairly clean-cut young man ... not necessarily your typical asker. He said he was collecting money so he could get back home to Manitoba. He said he came to Vancouver to live for a short time and ran out of money and he couldn't get a room in a hostel or at the Salvation Army because of the dog he acquired on his travels—his new best friend. He proceeded to tell me his life story while I sat on the sidewalk beside him and petted his dog.

He definitely had had some struggles throughout his young life and not much support, not a lot of love. He told me he accepted Jesus at one time, but veered off that path and got a little lost. He told me he even had a small Bible at the bottom of his bag somewhere, but he never read it.

I remember I didn't have much cash on me that day ... I had two fives or two tens—I gave him one of the bills and a granola bar or chocolate bar or something, and I left. I got a few blocks away as I headed toward Granville Street and had the urge to turn back and take him the other bill I still had in my wallet. I tried to ignore the inner voice telling me to go back, because I wanted to get on with my walk, plus, I thought I might need that bill ... I was getting hungry.

Like many other times, I lost the argument with the inner

voice and I went back. When I reached my new friend and his dog, I was happy to see him reading his Bible and he was happy to see me with more money. And I just ate lunch when I got home.

Anyway, had I not been struck by lightning that day and had my closed mind stayed that way, I would have missed out on an opportunity to give and I would have missed out on an opportunity to receive. All I gave was my lunch money, but what I received was understanding and wisdom, which is, of course, invaluable.

A dog's love is like God's love—it's accepting, it's enduring, it's unconditional. A dog loves you regardless of what you look like, regardless of your age, your race, your gender, your occupation, your potential earning capacity. This dog and most dogs love the rejected, the homeless, the broken, the beggar, the sick, the sinner.

We all need this kind of love ... it's what we look for, it's what we long for. The guy on the street is just like the woman at the well ... we all are! The woman at the well was thirsty; she was looking to quench the thirst of her soul ... to be made whole. The woman at the well was a Samaritan woman, and Jewish people didn't speak to Samaritans; but Jesus did. When Jesus met the Samaritan woman at the well, to quench her spiritual thirst, He told her that He could give her living water. Jesus said, "Everyone who drinks this water will be thirsty again, but whoever drinks the water I give them will never thirst. Indeed, the water I give them will become in them a spring of water welling up to eternal life," (John 4:13-14).

Understandably, she didn't get it. When He told her to go get her husband and come back, she said she didn't have one. He told her that she was right and that she had had five husbands and the man she was with now was not her husband. Jesus met her that day with all the right answers and the ability to quench her thirst for a love no other man could offer.

"For God so loved the world that He gave His one and only Son, that whoever believes in Him shall not perish but have eternal life."
John 3:16

Stormy Weather—March 7, 2013

The sun came out on Sunday. It was so exciting, I felt like a kid on Christmas morning. Everyone was smiling; it was like we'd all won the lottery. That might sound a little exaggerated, but after days of torrential downpour and months of grey clouds and rain, a day of sunshine can change your life. Our town, Maple Ridge, is also known by the locals as "Rainy Haney."

Haney was the original name of the downtown core of Maple Ridge, named after Thomas Haney, one of the first settlers. Vancouver and area, including Vancouver Island, has the mildest winters of all of Canada, but the wettest. Those of us drowned rats in Rainy Haney are convinced we are the most soaked; I guess you could say, we're all wet. The mountains we are nestled up against and the rivers that run through our community are contributing factors.

The rain starts early in the fall and by February, gathering pets and building an ark come to mind. In the spring when we all crawl out from under our umbrellas, we rejoice and agree we live in a special place. Intermittent showers continue throughout the spring and summer, but like Mike always says, "What do you expect? We live in a rain forest."

On sunny Sunday, Mike and I went for a three-and-a-half-hour walk. We walked to Erin's and she joined us on our walk to town. We walked and talked and soaked up the warm rays of the sun. It was glorious! We also spent time chatting in the park. Erin told me to have a seat on a bench and she stood behind Mike and gave him a shoulder massage. We had a great time; it was just what the doctor ordered, including a desperately needed dose of vitamin D.

The sun shone on Monday as well ... bonus, two sunny days in a row! But even though the sun was shining outside, there was a storm brewing inside me. Mike had home care and I had plans to meet a friend for a coffee and then run some errands; but, out of nowhere, the guilt hit me like a ton of bricks ... grief and guilt. Grief from the losses, and guilt because I *can* go out; I can drive and walk and talk with a friend on a beautiful day and Mike can't. Plus, I really miss Mike when we are apart. It's like a tug of war in my heart; I don't want to go out and leave Mike behind, but I know I have to get out sometimes; I need a break, because I have "Caregiver Burnout," which I recently researched at the prompting of Mike's respirologist. I learned from the respirologist, who was acting more like a psychologist, about caregiver burnout and it seems I have most of the symptoms.

I guess she could see through me at Mike's last appointment. She spent five minutes explaining Mike's lung function based on his latest tests, and about twenty-five minutes talking about the importance of me being Mike's wife first and not his number one caregiver. Holding back the tears, I kept smiling, and in my head I was thinking, How on earth can I do that? By God's grace, I am both; I have been able to be his primary caregiver and still have a loving and passionate relationship with him. She talked about the guilt I was probably experiencing, because I wasn't given a death sentence, and Mike has been. She called it "Survivor Guilt" and she hit the nail on the head with that one. She also told Mike that he would experience guilt, because he probably feels like he is holding me back from growing as a person and moving forward with my life.

I knew she knew what she was talking about, but I was thinking, How on earth can I grow as a person and move forward with my life when Mike and I are one? We have been married for almost twenty-five years and it's perhaps impossible for us to go in different directions. I must admit, something in me says, "Live!" but I don't want to without him. And so the storm in me roared.

In my last blog post, "Golden Boy," I said that we are all in the same boat; we all experience troubles of many kinds. Since then I keep thinking about a boat story from the Bible. Luke 8:22-25 says, "One day Jesus said to his disciples, 'Let us go over to the other side of the lake.' So they got into a boat and set out. As they sailed, He fell asleep. A squall came down on the lake, so that the boat was being swamped, and they were in great danger. The disciples went and woke Him, saying, 'Master, Master, we're going to drown!' He got up and rebuked the wind and the raging waters; the storm subsided, and all was calm. 'Where is your faith?' He asked his disciples. In fear and amazement they asked one another, 'Who is this? He commands even the winds and the water, and they obey him.'"

When I got home from my outing on Monday, with a big smile on his face, Mike asked how my time out was. I am probably the only one who could have understood him with his impaired speech. And he is probably the only one who could have understood me when the floodgates I was desperately trying to contain burst open as I explained that I missed him so much.

Well, today is Thursday and it's raining again, but the storm in me has subsided. I called on the Lord and boy, am I glad we're in the same boat! I suspect there will be more storms, but I'm going to cling to the One who even the winds and waters obey.

Savour the Moment—March 18, 2013

I was exhausted this morning when the alarm went off at 7:00 a.m. I tried to get to bed at a decent time last night, but that didn't happen and I knew I was going to pay for it this morning. On Sunday nights, we have been watching the miniseries, *The Bible*, which is fantastic and then Mike has been watching *Vikings* after that from 10:00 to 11:00 p.m. Then it's the big push to get to bed. I crush up his meds and feed those to him in yogurt. Then I brush his teeth and wash his face and then transfer him from his chair to his wheelchair. I then wheel him to the bedroom, transfer him to the edge of the bed, take off his shirt, give him a good back scratch, and then swing him up on the bed. Then I take off his shoes and socks and arrange all of his pillows where he likes them and then turn him on his side. I get his arms where he wants them and put on his hand braces. That is about a thirty-minute process.

Going to bed right after would have been wise, but I stayed up to check my emails, so I didn't get to bed until about 12:15. I remember looking at the clock at 12:22 a.m., when I was finally tucked in. At 12:45, Mike wanted to turn over. At 1:15, he had to go pee and at 2:30, he needed to turn over again. Needless to say, when my alarm went off at 7:00 a.m., I laid there for a while, talking myself out of rolling over and going back to sleep.

In order to get to the Step Interval class I teach on Mondays in time at 9:00 a.m., I have to get Mike up by 8:00. I get him up and out to his chair and give him a little bit of breakfast through his feeding tube. I brush his teeth and make sure he is comfortable. I have to get his laptop in the right place so his one knuckle can click the mouse. Believe it or not, that can sometimes take a few minutes. I put on a TV show or some music, then I fly out the door.

Yesterday morning, I subbed a class for a fellow instructor who was sick. It was a 10:00 a.m. class, so that gave us a little more time to get up and ready. The day before that, Saturday, Mike stayed in bed while I went and taught my 9:00 a.m. Step class. Sometimes, Mike stays in bed in the morning while I go to my class and then I get him up when I get home between 10:00 and 10:30. He has been doing this a little more often lately and I think it's good, because I've noticed his best sleep is from about 5:00 to 10:00 a.m.

Anyway, on Saturday after my class, I headed straight back to bed when I got home. It was pouring rain and I was feeling the chill after my workout, so I thought I would snuggle in against my husband's hot body. Mike is really warm-blooded and I am usually cold, so stealing some heat from him is common for me.

After taking off his hand braces and removing some pillows, I nuzzled my way in there the way our little kitten, Professor Fluffy, used to nuzzle her way in under the blankets and into my arms on a cold morning … I think I was purring too, like she did. It reminded me of what we had, when Mike would wrap his arms around me and pull me close. I took his hand and slowly pulled back his fingers and pressed his palm up against mine. For half a minute, I forgot about ALS. We listened to the rain, the illness disappeared, and I savoured the moment.

I've been thinking about *The Bachelor* Finale that was on TV last week. I'm not a huge fan of the show, but sometimes I tune in for the last four episodes. I'm only interested in who the Bachelor or Bachelorette has narrowed it down to and I particularly liked Sean Lowe; he was super cute and seemed like a really nice guy. The finale dilemma is that some unlucky lady goes home with a broken heart and the other gets the knight in shining armour and a shiny rock for her finger. While Sean was proposing and his elated fiancé to be was quickly finding her way to cloud nine, they talked about their future and how they couldn't wait to get started with their lives together, and eventually grow old together. They mentioned growing old together a few times. It was a beautifully romantic scene and I'm sure most viewers would have been swept away.

We all talk about growing old with the one we love, and we make plans. Mike and I had plans to snuggle together in bed on rainy Saturday mornings for years to come, but now we just live for each day and are grateful for the moments we can still savour.

> *"Why, you do not even know what will happen tomorrow. What is your life? You are a mist that appears for a while and then vanishes. Instead, you ought to say, 'If it's the Lord's will, we will live and do this or that.'"*
> **James 4:14-15**

I don't teach a class tomorrow morning, so "Lord willing," Mike and I will spend a little more time under the covers and I will put my cold hands and feet against his hot body and he won't mind—he likes to keep me warm.

The Writing on the Wall—April 5, 2013

I remember it like it was yesterday. Mike came out of the men's washroom with a mischievous grin on his face. It was one of those "I'm up to something" grins that I had seen many times before. Erin, Karen, my mom, and I were waiting for him in the hall of the Science wing of the Education building at UBC. We were there for an event Erin's class was hosting, about eighteen months ago.

Mike wanted a pen—he didn't tell us why he wanted a pen— but he needed a pen. We all checked our purses and pockets— no pens. He would accept any writing instrument: a felt pen, a pencil, a crayon, an eyeliner, whatever we could offer. I had a lipstick, but I needed to know what it was for. With the same grin he had when he came out of the washroom, he ushered me in. He pointed to the writing on the wall in one of the washroom stalls. It said, "God is dead—Nietzsche."

Mike is pretty passionate about his beliefs and needed to respond to set the record straight. As much as I opposed the idea of my expensive lipstick being used to write the rebuttal on the wall in the men's washroom stall, I didn't really have a choice. It was Mike's duty to make right the wrong of a student who was long gone, for the sake of every other student yet to use that toilet. So I handed over my lipstick and Mike made the necessary changes. Now, written in larger letters on the wall of the stall in L'Oreal's Mulberry (a creamy plum with a hint of pink), it says, "Nietzsche is dead! God is alive!"

Having just celebrated Easter, the death and resurrection story is still resonating in my mind. The picture of a beaten and bloodied Jesus and His brutal death on the cross leaves me speechless, humbled, and extremely grateful. He paid a huge price as God's sacrifice, nailed to a wooden cross, along with the sins of the whole world. Not only did Jesus die for mankind, He rose again. It's the greatest victory in all of history and our God lives!

"For the wages of sin is death, but the free gift of God is eternal life in Christ Jesus."
Romans 6:23, NLT

Considering gifts are usually free, "free gift" is a little redundant, but I guess the word "free" in this New Living Translation of the Bible is used to stress the point that the price has been paid, and there is nothing we can do or have to do to earn a place in God's kingdom. You must believe in Him to receive the prize, but the cost is covered.

Oswald Chambers says, "The underlying foundation of the Christian faith is the undeserved, limitless miracle of the love of God that was exhibited on the Cross of Calvary; a love that is not earned and can never be."

Who doesn't like free stuff? I love free stuff! But we're talking about a home in heaven here, not a free sample at the grocery store or a buy-one-get-one deal on shoes. This is big ... it's huge ... it's everything!

Over the years, Mike has often quoted the wise and famous words, "The best things in life are free." After a walk on the Sea Wall in Vancouver or a bike ride on the dike here in Maple Ridge or a picnic in the park or at the beach, Mike, with a big smile on his face would remind me and the kids that indeed, the best things in life *are* free! The best things *beyond* this life are free too. And Mike, closer to the "beyond," is drawing strength and encouragement from his "free gift" of eternal life.

When I asked Mike the other night why he rarely gets down and is never depressed, he explained, "I've got my eyes on the prize!"

The following is a prayer similar to the one Mike and I prayed at different times in our lives when we decided to follow Jesus and accept God's free gift of eternal life:

> *"Lord Jesus, Thank You for dying on the cross for my sins and rising again to give me eternal life. Please forgive my sins. I open the door of my heart and receive You as my Lord, Saviour and Friend. Thank You for forgiving my sins and for giving me new life. Help me to trust in You and follow You from now on. Amen!"*

~ ~ ~ ~ ~ ~ ~

When I wrote, "The Writing on the Wall," I added the prayer in there at the end last minute. I thought perhaps someone reading might be interested in receiving this "free gift" for themselves. You never know who might be "seeking" and wanting exactly what you have. Calling out to God in repentant faith is the first principle of Christianity and the above sample prayer is a way to do that and begin a personal relationship with Him.

My sister and I were taught when we were teenagers to be prepared to share what we believe. My dad took us to seminars on how to share our faith; he later led his own seminars. I wasn't really into it as a teenager; but as an adult, I was glad to have the learning. I remember once going door to door, with a few others, to talk to people about God. It was probably the last thing I wanted to do on a Saturday afternoon. I was nervous and a little embarrassed, but that kind of stuff builds character, and here I am today sharing my faith ... I guess you could say this is my way of going door to door.

The Gospel Message ("gospel" means the teaching or revelation of Christ; the good news) can be narrowed down:

God loves you and wants you to experience His love, His peace, and His plans for your life.

Our sin separates us from knowing God, His love and His peace and plans.

Jesus came to atone for our sins and bridge the gap between us and God.

Our response—We must receive Jesus as Lord and Saviour to experience freedom from sin, a relationship with Him, and assurance of a home in heaven. It's not supposed to be complicated like religion sometimes is ... it's about relationship.

I can't imagine my life without this relationship!

"To be loved by God is the highest relationship, the highest achievement, and the highest position in life."
Henry T. Blackaby

It's All Relative—April 28, 2013

Madison is home. First year university, accomplished! It was a tough year, but she did it and we are really proud of her. Madison wasn't happy being away from her family. And when she left for university last August, we were packing up the family home; our house was sold and we had already moved to my sister's house. Plus, we were looking for new homes for her beloved pets: her cats, Professor Fluffy and Pepsi, and her dog, Molly. I can't imagine how tough that was for her.

It was love at first sight when Madison found Molly online. Madison searched for the perfect pooch after grieving the loss of her first dog, Isla. Mike couldn't understand why we would go to Bellingham, Washington to adopt a dog. He kept asking why we would go to the United States for a dog, when there was a perfectly good pound just a few miles away. He stopped asking when we brought Molly home and he met our adorable new puppy for himself ... and fell in love.

Madison was only a few weeks away from finishing her first year of university when she surprised us and came home for the Easter long weekend. She caught a ride with some friends and showed up wearing blue bunny ears and carrying a basket of chocolate. It was a wonderful surprise and on the second day of her three-and-a-half-day visit, Nathan came over and said he was going to call Christian and arrange a visit with Molly.

Christian is Nathan's friend. They became friends in grade eight and one day shortly after, they figured out that they were cousins as well ... kind of. Christian was over at our house and saw a picture on the fridge and asked Nathan why we had a picture of his cousins on our refrigerator (a Christmas picture of my cousin Sean's children). Nathan told him that they were *his* cousins. Turned out that Nathan and Christian had the same second cousins through the marriage of his great-aunt Marguerite (my mom's sister) and Christian's mom's uncle Trevor (her dad's brother).

Tragically, Uncle Trevor died in a plane crash many years ago when their fourth child and only girl was just a baby. Now, their three sons and daughter are in their thirties and forties and have beautiful families of their own ... Uncle Trevor would be extremely proud!

Anyway, Molly lives with Christian and his mom and dad, Alison and Raj and brother Taylor. The Hardie family is Molly's new family and Nathan felt it was time Madison (and Mike and I) saw Molly; it had been way too long since our last visit.

When Nathan hung up with Christian, he said, "Let's go!" and we were off to see Molly.

Molly was happy to see us, but it was apparent, she was a full-fledged Hardie. They were her people now and she loved them the way she loved us when she lived at our house. And the Hardies love her. Molly is their dog now and we are really happy for all of them.

Shortly after Molly moved in with the Hardies, in a message from Raj, he said, "Molly has been a blessing. A smile that's been missing from our faces since our Golden Retriever Max died."

It's a unique friendship for sure. Not only do we share the same relatives, we share the same love for a wonderful dog. But even more than all that, we share the same illness: ALS. Alison's dad had ALS.

One day not long ago, Alison sent me a lovely message, including three poems her mom wrote years ago. I was overcome with emotion, because reading the poems was like reading a portion of my own heart. I didn't know Alison's mom, Judy (though, I might have met her when I was a child), but now I feel I know her well.

With permission from Alison, here are Judy's poems.

May 15—Me

A brave façade.
A stiff upper lip.
I am tough and I keep my pain well hidden.
But the smallest of things reveal my fragile self.
My body betrayed with unexpected tears.

A kind word.
A remembered melody.
The sound of a bird in the morning.
There should be joy in the morning.

May 26—We

Last night I held you.
I ran my hands over your back; your body is frailer now.
No, frail is not the right word … less robust.
I saw the obscene twitching of nerves on your back
And know it is spreading when you touch me.
Your fingertips are cool, your touch so delicate,
But I know this is the new you.
And can you still feel me?

July 23—Going Backwards

You walk unsteadily carefully planting.
One foot before the other.
You eat uncertainly, grasping with difficulty the fork and the
spoon.
You speak haltingly each word carefully chosen:
Simple, monosyllabic.
You cry unabashedly.
Heart on sleeve.
At a moment's whim.
Body behaving like a child's.
Heart and mind: still you.

Alison went on to say in her message:

"A month later, my mum was diagnosed with Ovarian Cancer so the battle spread to two fronts.

"Anyway, I am sharing this with you because I appreciate that you are sharing your experiences. I think it helps everyone to understand the disease, but most importantly you are allowing God's grace to shine in your lives."

John lived with ALS for less than a year. He died in 1997 and Judy died three years later.

Turning Over a New Leaf—May 8, 2013

Mike put on his Leaf's T-shirt this morning in anticipation of the NHL play-off game against the Boston Bruins tonight. The Bruins are ahead of the Toronto Maple Leafs, two games to one of the best-of-seven-games series, but Mike is hopeful his team is going to tie it up. Mike is a faithful fan and an optimistic one as well.

Yesterday when he woke up, he told me he thought the Canucks would make a comeback and win the game and go on to win the series. The Vancouver Canucks were of course down three games to none (also the best-of-seven-games series) against the San Jose Sharks and many of their fans were calling them a bunch of bums already, but not Mike. He hasn't said a negative word and when the game started, he was wide-eyed, cheering on the inside.

Unfortunately, Mike's prediction was incorrect and the Canucks lost the game in overtime. Mike was close though. He had a vision earlier in the day that the game would go into overtime and Daniel Sedin would score. The game did go into overtime, but Daniel Sedin ended up in the penalty box and the Sharks scored. Mike cheered for them to the very end and was pleased they played well.

I have proudly written about Mike's incredibly positive attitude many times, but Mike is human and he fell into a little slump last week. It's unusual for Mike to be down, but it's understandable for sure. Once in a while, I think he just needs to grieve what's gone, while 99 percent of the time, he is happy, content, and thankful for what he has. I noticed it on Wednesday and by Saturday Mike was still not himself.

Nathan went to Kelowna for the weekend to play in an Ultimate Frisbee Tournament, so Leah stayed with us. She came on Friday and having her over definitely helped, but Erin, Madison, and I continued to work together to cheer Mike up.

Mike and I had plans to meet his good friends, Dan and Ron, at the local casino to watch the Kentucky Derby horse race on Saturday afternoon. It's a tradition for Mike and these long-time buddies to watch the famous race together.

The three men always got together a few times a year to go to the races, or a hockey game, or out for a burger and a beer. They love to talk about events at Riverview Hospital where they all worked at one time, or the games of ball hockey or slow pitch when they played on the same teams. Nothing causes their bond to become stronger than recalling fond memories, including past races won, remembering the names of the horses with smiles on their faces ... Charlie's Pride, Lucky Lady, Warm Annette ... and now Ron's pick, number 16, Orb, who won the big race this year.

I was really hoping Mike's horse would win to help cheer him up. Mike's horse started well, but landed somewhere in the middle of the pack. My two-dollar win-place-and-show bet on number 4, Golden Soul, made me fifty bucks richer and, like the couple of other times I've placed a bet and won, I stopped while I was ahead.

Erin and Madison took Leah out so Mike and I could meet Ron and Dan. Mike was happy to see his good buddies, but I knew he wasn't necessarily in the mood for the horse race. Mike always liked to study the racing program; he liked to do a little research on the horses running in the race and converse with the guys about the jockeys and the condition of the track etc., but Mike can't do that anymore and it was disappointing.

Mike and I left the casino right after the race. We walked over to the park across the street and spent some time there being disappointed. Alone together on a beautiful day in the shade, in a quiet place, to breathe, to grieve for a few minutes, and then, onward!

We had asked Erin and Madison to bring Leah and meet us at the little pottery place on Dewdney Trunk Road so Leah and I could work on a project for Mother's Day. Erin and Madison took Mike for a walk while Leah and I got creative.

I was glad for Mike, because I knew Erin and Madison would take Mike back to the park, entertain him with witty banter, and give him a head and neck massage (Erin's famous head rub).

When Leah and I were finished our project we went to meet them and the "three amigos" met us with three large grins and a picture. The two girls managed to get Mike in the photo booth at the mall … I don't know how they did it and I can't believe they did it, but they did it, and they were proud of their accomplishment and had a priceless souvenir.

By the end of the day, Mike's smile was back and he seemed himself. Wide-eyed and cheering on the inside, he watched his team; the Leafs beat the Bruins that night and all was right.

Tonight's game is another nailbiter. I finish this blog post during the second intermission of the Leafs game. It's tied, 3-3. I'm also cheering on the inside for Mike's team ... "Come on boys win another one for my guy Mike. He is one of your biggest fans!"

> *"Perseverance means more than endurance—more than simply holding on until the end. A saint's [Christian's] life is in the hands of God like a bow and arrow in the hands of an archer. God is aiming at something the saint cannot see, but our Lord continues to stretch and strain, and every once in a while the saint says, "I can't take any more." Yet God pays no attention, He goes on stretching until His purpose is in sight and then He lets the arrow fly. Entrust yourself to God's hands!"*
> **Oswald Chambers**

Keep Smiling—May 22, 2013

Madison had a great game Sunday night. She scored a couple of goals and had lots of energy. The whole team played really well.

Her team, "Moose on the Loose," is an all-girl, 3-on-3 ice hockey team. They play in a co-ed spring hockey league every year after the regular ice hockey season is over. With only three players on the ice at a time plus the goalie, it's fast. The girls say it's super fun and a great workout!

Most of their competitors are boys. The girls don't beat the boys as much as they used to; the boys are young men now and are much bigger and stronger than they were a few years ago; but regardless, the girls always give the boys a run for their money. Last game was no exception. The boys beat the girls, but not by much and not without a good fight.

From the end of the first period until we left the rink, Mike had a smile on his face that wouldn't quit. I commented on his contagious smile while we were getting him in the car. He didn't say a word, he just smiled bigger.

It's a huge process getting Mike in and out of the car; we don't go out in the car very often. It takes a team. Madison and I did the lifting and lowering and positioning, and my parents helped with taking the wheelchair apart and fitting it all in the trunk like puzzle pieces. Mike just smiled the whole time.

Earlier that day, I watched Mike watch Erin read Leah a book. It was a French book and Erin read the book to Leah in her usual enthusiastic way, and Leah watched and listened as though she could understand every word. Mike watched and smiled. It was that same smile that said, "I am thoroughly enjoying myself." It also spoke of being proud, happy, and thankful.

Mike has a great smile. It was one of the things that attracted me to him right away. He has no idea how his smile has impacted my life all these years. It has encouraged me, it has inspired me, and it has comforted me. When he smiles at me, it makes me feel really good and I can't help but smile back. His smile is like a reward. It's a special gift. It's a warm and wonderful gesture of love. And now, when words are few, I appreciate his smile more than ever.

ALS has taken so much, but Mike's smile is still intact and I am thankful!

Fear Less—June 6, 2013

This blog post is dedicated to our children, Erin, Nathan, and Madison, and to our granddaughter, Leah. I encourage you to put your faith before your fears and never let anything stop you from being all you are meant to be, from doing all you are supposed to do, and from experiencing God's very amazing and wonderful plans for your lives. And to my parents and my sister for their endless prayers and for helping me to face my fears.

I woke up early this morning—about 5:00 a.m. Newfoundland and Labrador time.

Mike went back to sleep after I helped him turn over, but I couldn't. I lay in bed and prayed for a while, and then got my cell phone and listened to some music. I just love this new rendition of an old hymn I have been listening to: "His Eye is on the Sparrow," written by Civilla D. Martin and Charles H. Gabriel in 1905. Yancy, the current artist, sings it beautifully on her new album, *Roots for the Journey*. The tranquil sound is lovely and the words are a wonderful reminder that God is near and He always takes care of us.

Before we left for the East Coast, I'd called upon some friends to pray for us; for Mike, yes, but mostly for me. It sounds selfish, but I am afraid of flying and rely on the prayers of family and friends to help me. I haven't always been afraid of flying, but I can't really remember when the fear first came knocking. I have been flying since I was young; trips to visit grandparents and aunts and uncles and cousins in Steinbach, Manitoba, a trip to Disneyland, and my first trip to Brazil when I was eighteen. Since then, I have flown many times: in Canada, trips to Calgary, Saskatoon, Winnipeg, Toronto, Ottawa, and short flights throughout BC; then there have been flights to Mexico, Brazil, Nigeria, Malawi, The Dominican Republic, Bulgaria, the US, and connecting flights throughout the US, Africa, and Europe. It's a lot of flying for someone who is afraid.

I hate saying I'm afraid, because the Bible says that, "Perfect love casts out all fear." Perfect love comes from my Heavenly Father whose perfect love I have known all my life. So why am I afraid? I have asked myself that question numerous times. I tell people, "I'm not afraid of dying, I'm just afraid of flying." I'm not afraid of the dark, I'm not afraid of heights (maybe a little sometimes). I'm not afraid of speaking in public. I wonder if the Lord allows this fear in my life to test my faith.

Elanna says that it is commendable that I don't let the fear stop me from flying. Family vacations, trips to visit friends and family and orphans in Africa, hockey tournaments, mission trips, Mike's medical treatments, new places, new faces, and all the amazing adventures have forced me to put my faith before my fear and it's one of the hardest exercises I have had to perform.

Joel Osteen says, "When fear comes knocking, let faith open the door." When I am all buckled up and the engines start to roar and the air plane jets down the runway and the front end lifts off the ground, my heart pounds and sweat beads—I am a nervous wreck. The fear knocks and my faith reluctantly opens the door and I rise above, visualizing God's big hand holding me up.

And so it is with ALS. We rely on God's big hand to hold us up. In order to enjoy the time we have left, we must let faith answer when fear knocks. Mike's strong faith and lack of fear encourages me every day!

I can't imagine my life had I let my fears ground me. Even still after every flight, I think perhaps it's the last one. But no, my faith is much greater than my fear and I look forward to my next adventure.

> *"God has not given us a spirit of fear and timidity, but of power, love and self-discipline."*
> **II Timothy 1:7, NLT**

So, to our dear children, and everyone: The Lord cares for the birds of the air, and how much more does He care for you. "So don't be afraid; you are worth more than many sparrows." Matthew 10:31.

Chapter 13
The Iron Horse

Spelling It Out—June 26, 2013

Mike hasn't been sleeping that well since we returned home from Newfoundland and Labrador. The trip was amazing and we had a great time visiting Mike's family in Toronto first, then seeing the sights of St. John's with my sister and watching Madison play ball hockey and win a gold medal, but the trip was exhausting for us. I knew it was going to be a challenge, but I also knew it would be worth it.

Mike slept well for the first time on Sunday night, but woke me early Monday morning. It was about 5:30 a.m. and he definitely had something to tell me. Half asleep, I went through the list: "Is your head itchy?" as I scratched his head vigorously, my eyes still closed. "Your eyebrow?" and I scratched both eyebrows with one hand like I usually do just to make sure I get the right one. "Your ear?" and I moved the scratching to his ear. I asked him if he needed to go pee, if he wanted to turn over, if he was comfortable. With one eye half open, I rearranged his arm on the pillow and I fixed his fingers.

Then I listened.

Mike started spelling it out: H? Yes. E? No. A? Yes. T? No. P? Yes. P again? Yes. Y? Yes. It took a while to get the next five letters: A, N, N, I, V, but finally I clued in—HAPPY ANNIVERSARY was what he had to say.

June 24 was our twenty-fifth wedding anniversary. It was a lovely day. We received so many wonderful messages and cards from family and friends and Pat was here along with my family, which made it extra special.

When I was nineteen and newly married, I had no idea what I'd got myself into. Mike and I thought it was a great idea to run off and get married, but when the honeymoon was over, I wondered if perhaps we should have taken more time to think about it. After all, "till death do us part" is a pretty big commitment.

At that age, I had no idea what I wanted in a husband. I honestly never thought about it much; and there I was saying, "I do." I knew I loved Mike and I was naïve, so that was good enough. I learned over the years what I wanted in a husband and, thankfully, Mike had what I wanted. He was far from perfect and sometimes he drove me crazy; but ultimately he has shown me many qualities that make a great husband.

We don't have a perfect marriage, but we have a good one. At times, it was great. At other times, it was just okay, sometimes, it wasn't okay. But today it's this beautiful thing, it's precious.

Because we don't know about tomorrow, and because we don't expect to celebrate another anniversary together, we cherish this one so much. We cherish every day … every minute.

On Monday night, our anniversary night, after tucking Mike into bed, I lay beside him with my arm around him. I didn't say a word, I just held tight. I was overcome with emotion and held the moment as tightly as I held Mike. If I could have spoken, this is what I would have said: "Thank you for your utmost respect all the time. Thank you for making me feel smarter than I am and more beautiful than I ever could be. Thank you for the endless laughter. Thank you for making me feel taken care of, cherished, and loved beyond measure. And thank you for listening; you are an excellent listener! You are my best friend, a great lover, a wonderful father and granddad, a brilliant person, and an incredible man!"

If Mike could have spoken, he probably would have said, "Happy twenty-fifth anniversary. It's been the best twenty-four years of my life!" (Mike's ongoing joke as the first year was pretty rough … I personally think the first three or four were pretty rough.) And then we would have laughed out loud together.

P.S. When we arrived home from our trip to the East Coast, we had an incredible gift waiting for us (not necessarily an anniversary gift, just a gift)—a beautiful white, shiny, new wheelchair van from Mike's parents. A little bit of freedom goes a long way…it's life changing! We are so grateful!

Swing, Batter, Batter—July 15, 2013

Ron and Dan came over last week for a visit It's baseball season, so that was one of our topics of conversation. We talked about how well Mike's home team, the Toronto Blue Jays are doing. We discussed with excitement the Jays' recent eleven-game winning streak. We also discussed with excitement the good old days when we all played slo-pitch together. That's how I first met Ron and Dan years ago when Mike took me out to play slo-pitch with him on his co-ed slo-pitch team when we first started dating.

Slo-pitch is softball with a few minor differences. Softball was my sport. Boys played baseball and girls played softball, but I would just like to clarify that the ball isn't soft at all. It's bigger than a baseball, but when it's smacked directly at you when you are standing on the pitcher's mound, it's definitely not soft.

I played the game from the time I was ten years old until I was about twenty-three. I was a pitcher, or as one of my first coaches called me, I was "the shooter." My dad to this day still calls me "the shooter" sometimes, imitating my old coach and laughing. I smile because it's a fond memory. Coach Bob pacing back and forth, yelling, "You're the shooter! Come on shooter!" My parents and other parents and my teammates cheered me on.

I didn't have the fastest pitch, but it was pretty accurate. I loved pitching, it was fun and exciting. I played a few other positions, including outfield, but I don't think I could have been a fielder full time. Standing around waiting for the ball to come my way wasn't my idea of excitement. Batting, though, now that was exciting! I think the most fun part of the sport is running the bases. Stealing second was always my top priority, third was next and even home sometimes. I was a little greedy I guess, but when an error is made by the other team, giving you the opportunity to score, you go for it, and don't hesitate!

Running bases was Mike's specialty. His team called him "wheels," because he was so fast. I can still see him rounding second and sliding into third on a base hit, the infielders eating dust and the rest of us applauding.

I think the game of baseball (or softball or slo-pitch) is a lot like life. There are a lot of exciting moments, but for the most part it can be quite monotonous. It's about systems and routines and thousands of swings at different opportunities that "come down the pike." Every batter faces a curveball now and again. In the sport, a curveball can change the game and in life, a curveball can change everything.

On March 7, 2011, when our curveball, ALS, crossed the plate, everything changed. You see it coming and suddenly you start to shake in your boots. You lose all the confidence you had the last time you were up to bat. The stance you perfected after years of practice is lost and you find yourself on your knees begging for mercy.

The late, great New York Yankee, Lou Gehrig was diagnosed with ALS in 1939 at the age of thirty-six. Two weeks after the first baseman was diagnosed, he retired from Major League Baseball with twenty-three grand slams (home runs when the bases are loaded) under his belt. He was twice named American Leagues' MVP, six times World Series champion, seven times all-star, and the Triple Crown winner of 1934. With the same courage and poise he had every time he stood in the batter's box, he delivered a retirement speech to a jam-packed Yankee stadium. He started his speech by telling the crowd that he considered himself the luckiest man on the face of the earth. I'm sure Gehrig was overwhelmed by the support he received that day from his fans, friends, and family, and all the other Yankees, including teammates, Babe Ruth and Joe DiMaggio.

Lou was nicknamed "The Iron Horse" for his amazing streak of consecutive games (2,130, which held a record for fifty-six years), for being the first MLB player to have his uniform, number 4, retired, and for being elected into the National Baseball Hall of Fame in 1939.

The truth is ALS really sucks! More truth, I have almost lost my mind a few times and still could. Mike though, is mostly good. He remains content.

With one foot in the batter's box and one foot out, looking to my old ball coach Hawk (Bruce) for direction, I can hear him telling me to keep my eye on the ball.

Mike's eyes are still on the prize and mine have been wandering all over the place. I almost forgot the number one rule in the game, "Keep your eye on the ball" and I almost forgot the number one rule in my life, "Keep your eyes on God!"

Lou ended his famous speech by saying, "I may have had a tough break, but I sure have an awful lot to live for." Mike feels the same way! Lou passed away in 1941 at the age of thirty-eight, two years after he was diagnosed.

Jesus says: "I have told you these things, so that in Me you may have [perfect] peace *and* confidence. In the world you have tribulation *and* trials *and* distress *and* frustration; but be of good cheer [take courage; be confident, certain, undaunted]! For I have overcome the world. [I have deprived it of power to harm you and have conquered it for you.]" John 16:33, Amplified Bible (square brackets and italics in original).

Ahoy, Matey—July 23, 2013—By Mike Sands

Madison was recently invited to play for Team Canada at the world ball hockey tournament ... Nadine, Elanna, and I tagged along. The tournament took place in Newfoundland and Labrador.

Newfoundland and Labrador is the easternmost province in Canada. The Vikings discovered Newfoundland and Labrador in the eleventh century. It wasn't settled until John Cabot landed on it in the early 1600s. Cabot noted in his journal that as he lowered a bucket in the Grand Banks, instantly the bucket became full of fish. When word got back to Europe of this abundance of fish, many pulled up stakes and set sail for what Eric the Red had called "Vinland."

Newfoundland and Labrador has rugged terrain and harsh weather that is similar to parts of Ireland. Irish settlers felt at home on "the Rock" and were one of the few groups that remained. Newfoundland and Labrador has a distinctive Irish flavour to it that remains until this day.

Up until the early twentieth century, Newfoundland and Labrador's economy was centred around the fisherman. Back in the olden days, the occupation of a fisherman was one of the most dangerous ones around. Many harrowing tales have been related of men battling the rough seas in an effort to get their share of the bountiful haul that awaited them. Many a "b'y" came back a man. A common epitaph in cemeteries was "lost at sea." In the good ol' days, fishermen didn't have the luxury of advanced weather systems or radios. It was strictly "red sky tonight, sailors delight" as their only warning of inclement weather. If the sea didn't get them, they also had to worry about being crashed into the shores by torrential winds, rain, and waves. Lighthouses eliminated many of these disasters.

When we were in Newfoundland and Labrador last month, we visited some of these lighthouses. Plaques around the lighthouse grounds showed the evolution and historical significance of the lighthouse in Newfoundland and Labrador. The first lighthouses were bonfires on the ends of points at harbour entrances. Candles were used in the eighteenth century. By 1800, oil lamps were used. Whale oil was often used after a kill. Kerosene, which was invented by a Canadian in the 1840s, was used extensively in Canada after 1860, because it was cheap, reliable, and efficient. Electric lights came to lighthouses around the end of the nineteenth century.

The lighthouse remains a very important tool in the Atlantic region. It stands to reason that Newfoundland and Labrador, being the easternmost point in North America, would have frequent interactions with foreign sailing vessels. The following is one such interaction. This is an actual radio conversation (released by the chief of naval operations) of a US naval ship with Canadian authorities off the shores of what was then Newfoundland in October 1995.

Canadians: "Please divert your course 15° to the south to avoid a collision."

Americans: "Recommend YOU divert your course 15° to the north to avoid a collision."

Canadians: "Negative. You will have to divert your course 15° to the south to avoid a collision."

Americans: "This is the captain of a US naval ship. I say again, divert YOUR course!"

Canadians: "No, I say again, divert your course."

Americans: "This is the aircraft carrier USS Lincoln, the second largest ship in the United States Atlantic Fleet. We are accompanied by three destroyers, three cruisers, and numerous support vessels. I DEMAND that you change your course 15° north. I say again, that's one five degrees north, or counter measures will be undertaken to ensure the safety of this ship."

Canadians: "This is a lighthouse. It's your call."

When I was a kid growing up in the Toronto area in the 1960s and 1970s, I remember that Newfoundlanders, or "Newfies" as they were referred to back then, were always the butt of many jokes. These jokes were generally corny in nature: e.g. "Question: How did the first Newfie get to Toronto? Answer: He got a breakaway while playing ice hockey on the Saint Lawrence River. Question: And how did he get back? Answer: he was called offside." Or the one where you ask your friend, "Question: How do you keep a Newfie in suspense? Answer: I'll tell you tomorrow." In other parts of the world, these corny jokes centred around the nations of Poland, Ireland, or Scotland. In Canada, we picked on Newfoundland. I'm not sure why we chose Newfoundland over any of the other provinces to be the butt of our jokes.

Although Newfoundlanders were the butt of many jokes when we were kids, they played a very important role during the Second World War. Newfoundland (it didn't become Newfoundland and Labrador until 2001) was strategically located on the shores of the Atlantic Ocean. It was a strategic post that the allies used to fuel and launch aircrafts, destroyers, and submarines. It was also our country's first line of defence against any invasion from the German enemy.

One historic battle off the coast of Newfoundland that was related to me by an "old tar" while I was visiting Newfoundland and Labrador last month went as follows.

HMS Newfoundlander was approached by two German destroyers off the Grand Banks. As the destroyers approached, the captain hollered out, "Cabin boy, cabin boy, get me my red coat." After the *HMS Newfoundlander* took out the two German destroyers, the captain took off his red coat and handed it to the cabin boy to put away. One hour later, five German destroyers approached *HMS Newfoundlander* and again, the captain hollered out, "Cabin boy, cabin boy, get me my red coat." After the five German destroyers were sunk by *HMS Newfoundlander*, the captain again took off his coat and handed it to the cabin boy to be put away. This time, the cabin boy inquisitively asked, "Captain, why do you always order me to get your red coat whenever the enemy approaches?"

The captain replied, "Well, son, I like to wear my red coat, because if I'm ever bloodied during the battle, none of my crew will realize I'm hurt and that is good for morale." An hour later, fifteen German destroyers surrounded *HMS Newfoundlander*. As well, the German destroyers had ten Stuka dive bombers accompanying them. The captain yelled out, "Cabin boy, cabin boy, bring me my brown pants."

I was diagnosed with ALS in 2011. When someone tells you you've got three to five years to live, your fear instinct kicks into overdrive. Anyone who says they're not afraid when first diagnosed is just fooling themselves. Even General George S. Patton, who had ice in his veins when staring down his enemies, stated, "If we take the generally accepted definition of bravery as a quality which knows no fear, I have never seen a brave man." All men are frightened. The more intelligent they are, the more they are frightened. But you can't stay in fear mode forever; you have to go on living. Like the captain of the *HMS Newfoundlander* and so many of the seamen who stared death in the face while on the high seas, they had to carry on. "When you're going through hell, just keep going," was probably a motto many of these men swore by.

The secret to getting yourself through trying times is to get yourself in the right frame of mind. In *The Wizard of Oz*, the cowardly lion needed the Wizard to give him a medal in order to put him in the proper mindset to face his fears. I look to God to get me in the right frame of mind to face this dire diagnosis. In nautical terms, God is THE Lighthouse. When your boat is in trouble, you have to keep your eyes on the Lighthouse. The Lighthouse will make your path straight and lead you to a safe landing.

Eventually all bad things must come to an end. There is a rainbow at the end of the storm. The rainbow may not be a cure for ALS, or a sudden reversal of my symptoms. But if you have the belief, like I have the belief, that something grand awaits us after this life, then there is nothing to fear.

I remember watching the movie, *Gladiator*. In it, Marcus Aurelius, Emperor of Rome, played by Richard Harris, states, "Never let the future disturb you. You will meet it, if you have to, with the same weapons of reason which today arm you against the present." So I wait, knowing that my faith is being sure of what I hope for, to paraphrase Hebrews 11:1.

P.S. One last Newfie joke that I remember from when I was a kid: "Did you hear about the Newfie who was killed while ice fishing? Ya, he was run over by a Zamboni at centre ice of Maple Leaf Gardens." Corny, yes, but it brings a nostalgic smile to my face every time.

"I's the b'y that builds the boat, And I's the b'y that sails her. I's the b'y that catches the fish and brings them home to Liza," (traditional Newfoundland folk song).

~ ~ ~ ~ ~ ~ ~

Oh, how I love "Ahoy, Matey"! When Mike wrote this post I felt like I was given the greatest gift—him—the guy on the inside. I later mention in a blog post my love for this story and how getting a glimpse of what's on the inside of Mike is like hidden treasure revealed!

Mike's blog posts are always a big hit with my blog readers. His posts are the most read posts. I tell him, "You're the star … they like to hear from you!"

The High Road—August 11, 2013

There is a lot to learn from a person who is decreasing in his body and increasing in his soul. I wouldn't even know where to begin to explain what I have watched and learned from Mike in the past two-and-a-half years. I am observing a miracle unfold right before my eyes. As his health declines and things are supposed to be getting uglier, there is so much beauty.

The decline of Mike's health would cause one to think that ALS has got him beat, but in fact, Mike is beating ALS by creating something beautiful out of it.

The apostle Paul in Philippians 4:12, says: "I know what it is to be in need and I know what it is to have plenty. I have learned the secret of being content in every situation, whether well fed or hungry, whether living in plenty or in want." It's like Mike becomes more content with every loss. It's a supernatural process where he loses, but gains. He is confined on the outside, but absolutely free on the inside. He can't move, but is more alive than most healthy human beings.

Here is my dilemma—I feel like every day is a day closer to our parting, but every day is more beautiful than the one before. Sometimes, I don't know where the tears of sorrow and the tears of joy meet. They flow mingled down my cheeks together and I've never before been so happy and sad at the same time.

I'm sure Mike thinks he has nothing left to give, but his giving is greater than ever and his teaching more profound. He is in a place God wants us all. He is in a place of total reliance on Him, a place of complete surrender, and a place of being one hundred percent available to God.

Being in that place has made him an incredible example.

He perhaps would say he has had no choice, but he has had a choice. He has chosen the high road and is graciously allowing the Lord to do His mighty work in and through him, opening up a whole new world to the people around him of God's great power and love. God's grace and goodness flow mingled down all over us.

We have been living with my sister and family for a year now. We miss the home we had and the life we had, but consider this a very special time. Family is our greatest treasure here on earth and being with family is everything to us. Our children and granddaughter, our parents, our siblings (including in-laws), our nieces and nephews, aunts and uncles, cousins, and dear friends are what we treasure and thank God for every day.

Heaven Scent—September 17, 2013

Mike has always liked pudding, cooked pudding, not that instant stuff. He liked it as a child and he likes it just as much as an adult. He used to make it for our children all the time—it was a perfect after-school snack. He would time it just right so the pudding was warm when the kids walked through the door. That's the way he likes eating it … warm. He also likes the pudding skin, so he would pour the pudding on plates instead of in bowls in order to get lots of pudding skin.

Mike no longer eats the pudding skin. He chokes on the skin now. So when I feed it to him, I carefully peel the firm top layer of the warm pudding away and take the softer, creamy goodness underneath it. Mike eats pudding pretty much every day. It is the perfect consistency. Anything thinner, like soup, is too thin; it slips down his throat without warning or goes down the wrong way. Anything thicker is too difficult to swallow.

A few bites of mashed potatoes and gravy once in a while, a little applesauce here and there, a couple of spoonfuls of ice cream or soft cheese when he craves something savoury, and pudding; this is what he eats, and the poor guy struggles with these. The rest of his calories get mixed in a blender and go in his feeding tube, straight to his stomach. Mike is determined to eat, and even though he probably shouldn't, he isn't ready to abandon his taste buds quite yet, and I don't blame him.

Eating is one of the great pleasures in life, and good food is a wonderful gift and a tremendous blessing. So, of course losing the ability to eat is terrible. Mike is taking it quite well though. I ask him what he would like to eat and he gives me a "let me think about it" look, and then we both laugh. His favourite foods like pizza, steak, Fettuccine Alfredo, and BBQ ribs are a thing of the past and when we smell these foods, or see them or talk about them, the look on Mike's face would say he lost a good friend.

A few months ago, when Mike's food selection was becoming more and more limited and we were both becoming more and more disappointed, I would visualize a banquet table laid out for him in heaven. The table covered with the most mouthwatering dishes imaginable. If we saw a big, fat, juicy hamburger advertised on TV, I'd tell him that it was going to be at his "big feast" as well.

It was very appropriate that a sermon preached this summer by Pastor Brad was on this very subject. The sermon topic was hospitality, and Brad spoke a lot about the banquet table in heaven and he carefully described the scene in his usual compelling way. I loved hearing him describe the dinner, or "the party," as he put it. It helped with my vision of Mike's feast ... a meal fit for a king! And of course, much better, and far more important than the meal itself, is the presence of a King: Jesus Christ!

These are some of the sermon notes I scribbled down on a scrap piece of paper:

- "Feast" or "banquet" is mentioned in the Bible over one thousand times, along with "food" and "friends."
- Revelation 19 talks about the feast at the end.
- Luke 14 talks about the banquet in heaven.
- The invitation goes out to everyone ... all are welcome!
- Have you trusted in Jesus? Are you going to the party?
- Give your sin to Him and He will give you His salvation.

A couple of days later, Carol ended an email with Song of Solomon 2:4: "He has taken me to the banquet hall, and His banner over me is love." Wow, great friends think alike!

Anyway, back to earth. Here, it is the season of fall already. Summer is over now, but won't soon be forgotten. It was a beautiful summer! We experienced record heat and it was the driest summer in years. Our daily walks mostly took place in the evening when it was a bit cooler. Most nights, the aroma of BBQ filled the air. Mike and I both agree; it's surely the scent of heaven!

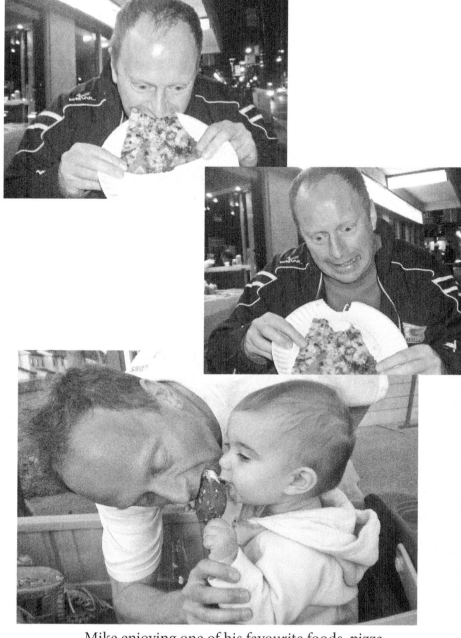

Mike enjoying one of his favourite foods, pizza,
and sharing ice cream with Leah.

Chapter 14
Double That and You Got Me

He is Able—September 24, 2013

When Mike was diagnosed with ALS two-and-a-half years ago, we prayed diligently for a long time that God would heal him. God didn't heal him, but He still could, and the decline of Mike's health doesn't make it more difficult for God to heal him now. God's power is limitless and it would be just as easy for God to heal Mike now as it would have been for God to heal him before the illness really took off.

I must admit though, my hope for healing faded a while ago and my prayers for healing waned. And then recently, God said to me "I am able!" And I said, "I know." And He said, "Then why don't you pray for your husband's healing anymore?" And then I asked for forgiveness and I asked for more faith. And then I resumed my plea!

It's funny, because hundreds of prayers have been answered since we first prayed for Mike's healing. But, why not this prayer? Why not the healing prayer?

I'm not really a "why?" person. I usually accept the "nos" with the "yeses," and trust God's decisions. And so it is with this as well. I have decided that I will pray for Mike's healing until it happens or until we part, and I'll continue to accept the "nos" with the "yeses," and praise God that He is able. And of course, I have to trust His decision.

Last night after I gave Mike his last smoothie of the day and crushed up his meds and put them in his feeding tube, I brushed his teeth, suctioned his mouth, washed his face, and stood him up; I held the urinal and he went pee. I gripped him really tightly around the backs of his arms and helped him inch his feet toward his wheelchair and I wheeled him to the bedroom. I parked him right beside his bed, suctioned his mouth again, stood him up, held him super tight, and helped him inch his feet to turn around and rest his butt on the edge of the bed. Then I flipped him onto the bed (I call the move "the flip"). I quickly made sure his arms were beside him comfortably and his head straight on the pillow. I took off his shoes and socks. I rolled him on his side and put a pillow behind him to keep him propped. I put a pillow between his legs, a pillow between his feet, a pillow under his top arm, and two small pillows stacked under his bottom arm, and I wrapped the fingers from both hands around the pillows. I pulled his shoulder out from under him slightly, tilted his head just a little, put an ankle brace on his left ankle, and suctioned his mouth again.

When Mike gave me his signature "good job" smile and in barely a whisper told me "perfect," I pushed my bed up against his bed, I ran to the washroom, I ran back, and I jumped in (Mike has been in a hospital bed for a couple of months now, so we sleep in separate beds … kinda like Lucy and Ricky Ricardo from the *I Love Lucy show*). Anyway, I jumped in and we said our prayers. I of course prayed for Mike's healing among many other things and praised God that He is able.

P.S. When Mike got his hospital bed, I slept on a mattress on the floor, intending to get a bed and just never got around to it. A few angels took care of it and got me a bed. I call the bed "the cloud," because it's so comfortable and because it came from three angels.

242

To the Moon and Back—October 5, 2013

A couple of weeks ago when I was at the grocery store, I picked up a jar of Smucker's® strawberry jam. I love Smucker's®, but I rarely buy it, because it usually costs more than all the other brands. While reaching for the less expensive and less tasty jam I normally buy, out of the corner of my eye, I caught a glimpse of the sale tag on the Smucker's®. No questions asked, I grabbed a jar and actually kind of hugged it. I grinned from ear to ear, not because of the dollar fifty in savings, but because the Smucker's® jam reminded me of Mike. When Mike did the grocery shopping, he didn't care about the price. He would get the Smucker's® because he knew I liked it best. And that is just one small way he showed his love.

Mike and I have had the same discussion regarding our love for each other many times over the years. It goes exactly like this: When he tells me he loves me, I ask him, "How much?" He shows me the distance of about an inch with his thumb and index finger.

I say, "That's it?"

He says proudly, "Compared to an ant!"

And then I say again, "That's it?"

He explains that, compared to an ant, an inch is a lot. He says that an ant can't even stretch his arms out that far as he stretches his arms out as far as he can.

I usually say one more time, "That's it?"

Then he asks, "Well, how much do you love me?"

I say, "To the moon and back compared to an ant." He replies, "Double that and you got me!"

Double? I don't think so, but maybe Mike has loved me

more than I have loved him. He was always thinking of me, always doing little things for me like writing notes for me on the dining room table with Alpha-Bits cereal, and he usually puts me first. He would probably say I did the same for him, but I just felt really loved. I still do, of course, even though he is unable to dump out a box of Alpha-Bits and construct "Mike loves Nadine" with the letters ... With a nod, a smile, and a certain look in his eyes, I know it's love.

Last weekend, Mike's health declined very quickly. Friday it started ... the coughing, gagging, choking, and by Saturday afternoon, we thought maybe it was pneumonia. We were constantly suctioning saliva from his mouth and trying different things to clear the congestion.

Saturday evening, completely exhausted and pretty much unable to breath, Mike agreed to go to the hospital. Elanna and I bundled him up, and we were off. Elanna drove and I sat in the back with my arms around Mike. We were all really calm on the outside, but on the inside I was pleading with God to give us more time. It seemed to happen so fast and I wasn't ready for this.

When we got to the emergency room of our local hospital, we were whisked in right away. Within fifteen minutes, Mike was having his chest X-rayed. Elanna and I were so surprised and really excited when the news came that his lungs were clear! His stats were great too! Like I keep telling Mike, he's the healthiest sick guy in town. Dr. Alan (a friend we were so happy to see), the nurse, and the respirologist were able to get things under control and in no time we were home again.

It's a week later and Mike is still fighting this nasty cold and, in his condition, it's pretty devastating. Throughout this whole ordeal, his gestures of love have been on my mind—the nod, the smile, the certain look in his eye, and all I can think is, "Double that and you got me!"

He'd reply, "Hey, that's my line."

After reading my recent blog post, "Heaven Scent," Mike's response was: "Man can't live on bread alone," from Matthew 4:4 where it says: "Jesus answered, 'It is written: Man does not live on bread alone, but on every word that comes from the mouth of God.'"

Mike hasn't eaten anything by mouth for a couple of weeks and he is still smiling ... wow!

Mike was given a medication to help dry up secretions. He tried the drops, but they weren't very effective, so he was prescribed the same medication to be injected. Elanna and I were given a lesson at the hospital, but the next day when I actually had to give Mike the injection and Elanna was at work, he coached me through it by typing step-by-step instructions on his laptop. When I was done, he typed, "Good job ... You are a natural ... I feel better already."

I left a bit of a welt, and it was red, but he just smiled.

In a Facebook message to me this week, Mike says, "I'm ready when He is."

"Courage is almost a contradiction in terms. It means a strong desire to live taking the form of readiness to die."
G.K. Chesterton

~ ~ ~ ~ ~ ~ ~

A few months after I posted "To the Moon and Back," my Uncle Larry showed up with a gift bag filled with jars of Smucker's® jam. He told me before he came he needed to drop off a "gift for me from Mike." I had no idea what he could possibly have for me from Mike and then I saw the jam ... I was so touched.

My Uncle Larry is one of those great men—salt of the earth types. I remember him well from when I was a little girl. He was so wonderful to be around ... he made me feel safe and he was fun. Now, he's still wonderful, still safe, and still fun. He has a great sense of humour, but he has a wonderful serious side that is wise and understanding.

We don't see each other a lot, even though we don't live far apart, but we stay in touch. We communicate by email mostly—on and off—and we get these discussions that go back and forth for a while sometimes. When Mike was diagnosed with ALS, I messaged my Uncle Larry ... and he of course was there for me. A couple of years before that, my Uncle Larry had a terrible back injury and was laid up for a long time while he waited for major surgery (he ended up having two surgeries). He lived with terrible pain for almost a year and was told he might not make a full recovery and may never play golf again. I remember the message after the long ordeal stating, "Our prayers were answered, I played golf today!"

We talk about our families, we encourage each other and exchange Bible verses and stuff like that. A lot of our conversations are long forgotten, but there is one discussion about some scripture I don't forget. The verse is Matthew 7:7, which says: "Ask and it will be given to you; seek and you will find; knock and the door will be opened to you." It's a verse I have always liked, but just happened to see it in a different light while we looked at it together.

I had read this verse many times before and always thought of it as a verse about getting prayers answered. And then I was struck, "Aha," it's about receiving, but not necessarily what you ask for.

This past spring, on June 9, I went to the dike on my bike.

It was the first time I had been to the dike without Mike since the last time we were there together months earlier. I was compelled to return, even though it was so painful. I sat on the bench where Mike and I always sat together and admired the Golden Ears Mountains, just like we always did. I was a little overcome with grief and then the Lord spoke to me, "Everyone who asks, receives …" And I had a wonderful time of prayer there. Later, I wrote in my journal, "When you ask, you come before God and there you receive … you don't necessarily receive what you ask for, but you receive all right … far more than you could hope for!"

Thrill Ride—October 28, 2013

Anyone who knows Mike well knows he's a big kid at heart. He has always loved pulling a good prank. He was quite often the instigator of neighbourhood water fights. He was "in there like a dirty shirt" when it came to a road hockey game. He's a die-hard trick-or-treater … which he and the kids are gearing up for in a few days. And he loved going to Playland.

Vancouver's Playland is the oldest amusement park in Canada and was one of our children's favourite places to go when they were younger. Sometimes, we all went as a family and sometimes, Mike would just take the kids and whatever friends wanted to tag along. Who better to take a bunch of kids to Playland than another kid, just bigger, with a driver's license and money, who rides all the rides and buys lots of mini donuts and cotton candy?

The park's main attraction and this family's favourite ride is the fifty-five-year-old wooden roller coaster. Simply named "the Coaster," this dangerous "thrill ride" isn't considered so because of its great height and super speed, but because it's "rickety" and without seat belts. The feeling of flying out of your seat at any moment is real and pretty scary, but hasn't happened to anyone ... yet.

ACE (American Coaster Enthusiasts) has honoured this famous roller coaster with "classic" and "landmark" status. ACE awards "landmark" status to rides that are historically significant and "classic" to wooden rides that use lap bars to allow the rider to float above the seat, have no other restraints so as to allow riders to move from side to side in the car, and a ride without head rests allowing all riders to view upcoming drops and turns.

All roller coasters have them ... drops and turns that is. They have their ups and downs for sure. The unexpected curves and swerves are all part of the ride. It can be exhilarating and terrifying! Life is kind of like that, too. It's a little hair-raising at times and can have you on the edge of your seat and sometimes you just want to scream, "GET ME OFF THIS THING!"

I'm not much of a thrill seeker myself. But when life feels like a wild ride, I find the best thing to do is to stay calm and trust God ... not necessarily in that order. Whether it's the twists and turns of ALS or anything else in our lives that seems a little over the top, I tell myself, STAY CALM AND TRUST GOD!

Some wise advice I applied to memory when I was young and I have been trying to apply to my life since then—a verse from Proverbs 3:5-6 that I have shared in my blog before—goes like this: "Trust in the Lord with all your heart and lean not on your own understanding; in all your ways, submit to Him [I learned it as 'acknowledge' Him] and He will make your paths straight." Memorizing and quoting this verse isn't that difficult, but putting it into practice can be. It's not something you learn to do in five minutes; it takes a lifetime to perfect.

My children know this verse well, or so they should. I've written it in birthday cards, I've spoken it on graduation day, I've sent it in Facebook messages. Last week, Madison and I were having a conversation via text messages. She was a little anxious as she contemplated big decisions. I texted "Don't worry AND trust God all the time."

She replied, "Okay."

I smiled and thought we should always respond that way.

Last week Mike and I prayed for friends who had to put their dog down ... a young man with a brain tumour ... a young friend with drug addiction ... a couple whose baby died ... friends with cancer ... friends with sick kids ... a mother's broken heart ... a friend with ALS ... one with Parkinson's ... other illnesses, alcoholism, depression, divorce, physical pain, and so on.

I'm sure we all feel like we are on a roller coaster ride sometimes. "Stay calm and trust God" should be written on the lap bar.

~ ~ ~ ~ ~ ~ ~

I remember thinking, when listing in "Thrill Ride" people we were praying for and their problems, "Wow, we don't have it so bad after all." Mike and I both agreed that ALS felt small next to the really tough stuff in other people's lives.

It felt even smaller when one of these friends died this past summer. After years of severe alcoholism, this beautiful fellow hockey mom succumbed. Her outer beauty long destroyed and her inner beauty long stolen by the demons that convinced her years ago it was the only way to cope.

She left behind three amazing daughters and a mom who had already lost her beloved husband, only son, and now her only daughter; this is tragedy. Life has lots of it. How do we respond ... how do we manage? It would be extremely insensitive to say to these girls and their grandmother, "Just trust God." But what do you say? You hope and pray they hang on for dear life and rise above the pain and strife, and strap on a life vest and cling to the One who can calm the winds and waters and the only One who saves us from a world of despair.

Grasping at Straws—November 13, 2013

Clean teeth and fresh breath have always been very important to Mike. Before he gave up control of his oral hygiene routine, he brushed, flossed, and rinsed with mouthwash a number of times a day. He carried dental floss with him in his pocket and kept some in the car. He would always take a step back when conversing with someone if he didn't think his breath was fresh. Same when I went in for a kiss, if he hadn't recently cleaned, he'd turn his head and give me his cheek instead of his lips.

I remember watching Mike brush his teeth with a hand that just wouldn't cooperate. He was losing the ability to hold his toothbrush and I knew he wasn't getting the cleaning he desired. But he kept doing the best he could and never gave up. He struggled for a while before I suggested I help. Without hesitation, he handed over his toothbrush. He didn't really have a choice; it was that or gingivitis. Plus, he was getting good at letting go.

Brushing Mike's teeth has become more and more of a challenge. He struggles to grip a straw with his lips and draw water up to his mouth. It can take a really long time, but Mike likes to rinse well before and after brushing. So, with the same persistence he has for so many other things, he keeps trying and doesn't give up. He is patient with himself. When water enters his mouth, he smiles a little. His lips, unable to seal tightly, allow some water to dribble out. After he swishes the water around in his mouth the best he can, he loosens his lips and the water spills out and rolls down his chin and I catch it in a dish. And then he repeats the process. He laughs at me sometimes, on my knees; I must look bored as I wait, but really I'm intrigued at his determination. My arms get tired holding the cup in one hand and the dish in the other. He probably thinks, "Some fitness instructor you are." He used to say that to me when I would cruise around a parking lot looking for the closest spot. When he drove, he always went straight to the back of the lot where there were lots of spots to park.

Anyway, Mike just never gives up. He doesn't quit. He has displayed the same constant determination at every stage of this illness without fail. Maybe sometimes on the inside he is screaming, but on the outside he is composed, calm, okay. He has had to let go of almost everything, but he still perseveres; he is still determined. He was once a strong, fit, athletic man capable of so much. Now with all his might, he draws water up a straw.

> "If God has made your cup sweet, drink it with grace; or even if He has made it bitter, drink it in communion with Him. If the providential will of God means a hard and difficult time for you, go through it ... You must go through the trial before you have any right to pronounce a verdict, because by going through the trial you learn to know God better. God is working in us to reach His highest goals until His purpose and our purpose become one."
> **Oswald Chambers**

~ ~ ~ ~ ~ ~ ~

I really like "Grasping at Straws." There are a few posts that are extra special to me and this is one of them.

I was asked by the ALS Society to write a story about Mike and our journey with ALS for a special promotion to raise awareness and money for the society. It was an article to be featured in the *Vancouver Sun* and the *Vancouver Province* newspapers. They asked me to write the story shortly after I wrote, "Grasping at Straws," so I included it in my piece, because it reveals what the illness was like for us right then.

The day the articles came out in both newspapers, Jamie from the ALS Society called and said that our story made a huge impact and donations were coming in, many in Mike's name. I remember exactly where we were on our walk when I received the call. Mike, Madison, and I were on Blackstock Street, walking by the tall trees—our favourite spot. Mike's face lit up when he heard he was instrumental in raising awareness and funds for ALS.

"Our spiritual life cannot be measured by success as the world measures it, but only by what God pours through us—and we cannot measure that at all."
Oswald Chambers

It wasn't long after I wrote, "Grasping at Straws" that Mike stopped taking water by a straw. Soon, the only water that went in his mouth was administered by a little sponge on a stick.

Take Hold of His Robe—November 21, 2013

A couple of weeks ago, feeling totally exhausted, completely drained, burnt out, and at the end of my rope, I called out to God (not out loud, just in my head) for a touch from His hand. There is power in His touch and I thought, if He would just reach down and touch me, I would have the strength to go on. A tap on the shoulder, a pat on the back, a kick in the pants …

any of those would do. If He would reach out and place His healing hands on me, I'd be okay. Almost instantly, after my quiet shout out to the Lord, I remembered another woman who was the epitome of someone totally exhausted, completely drained, burnt out, and at the end of her rope. A woman I read about in the Gospels and then really got to know and came to appreciate when I read the book *He Still Moves Stones* by one of my favourite authors, Max Lucado.

This is her story from Mark 5:24-34: "A large crowd followed Jesus and pressed around Him. And a woman was there who had been subject to bleeding for twelve years. She had suffered a great deal under the care of many doctors and had spent all she had, yet instead of getting better, she grew worse. When she heard about Jesus, she came up behind Him in the crowd and touched His cloak, because she thought, 'If I just touch His clothes, I will be healed.' Immediately her bleeding stopped and she felt in her body that she was freed from her suffering.

"At once Jesus realized that power had gone out from Him. He turned around in the crowd and asked, 'Who touched My clothes?'

"'You see the people crowding against You,' His disciples answered, 'and yet you can ask, 'Who touched Me?'

"But Jesus kept looking around to see who had done it. Then the woman, knowing what had happened to her, came and fell at His feet and, trembling with fear, told Him the whole truth. He said to her, 'Daughter, your faith has healed you. Go in peace and be freed from your suffering.'"

Max Lucado paints a very vivid picture of this nameless woman, who was at the end of her rope. He educates his readers, explaining that this situation would be very difficult for any woman at any time in history, but nothing could be worse for a

Jewish woman. She was considered unclean. She couldn't touch or be touched by her husband. She couldn't have children. She couldn't do household chores. She couldn't enter the temple.

She would have been completely exhausted, socially ostracized, probably friendless ... helpless ... desperate. Then comes a glimmer of hope—Jesus. Without any other options, she takes a chance and risks it all. Had she been recognized, big trouble. With no other choices, she pushes her way through the crowd, reaches out, and touches His robe. Instantly she's healed.

Occasionally I crash. Taking care of a man with ALS is a big job. It's sometimes too big. Even though we have excellent help, I burn out. Though mentally, physically, and emotionally spent, there is no "calling in sick" or "taking some holiday time." A couple of weeks ago, not able to even pray out loud, in my head and in my heart, I asked for a touch. And then this woman came to my mind and inspired me to reach out and touch Him. "Take hold of His robe," I have been repeating to myself since then ... "Take hold of His robe!"

Are you exhausted? Burnt out? At the end of your rope, perhaps hanging by a thread? Are you feeling helpless, hopeless, alone, afraid? Are you worried, sick, broke, or just simply broken? Take hold of His robe ... take hold of His robe!

P.S. I have had a few weekends away over the last year, thanks to the help of great home care staff and a wonderful team of family members, including Nathan who stays with Mike overnight and who is able to assist Mike with all his needs. Mike says Nathan is an excellent caregiver. I have a hard time leaving Mike for a few hours, let alone a couple of days, but I've learned that a little time away is beneficial for me and for everyone.

Chapter 15
Richie Rich

I had a friend named Richie—I called him Richie Rich. I first met him when I picked him up hitchhiking one day (picking up hitchhikers is not a common practice for me and I don't encourage it). I was running some errands after teaching a class one morning and I saw him in front of Greenwell Produce on Dewdney Trunk Rd. He had long white hair and a long white beard and he leaned on a long walking stick. When I drove past him, I noticed a toothless grin and I thought there was just something about him. I felt like I was supposed to give him a lift ... turned out he gave me a "lift."

I pulled into the store's parking lot and observed him from a distance for a little while. I called Mike and told him about this longhaired, gypsy-like old man. "I think I should pick him up. What do you think?"

"Yah, you should."

I joked and said, "Hopefully, I'll see you later."

Richie was so pleased when I pulled up. His toothless grin expanded and he was grateful I helped him get into my van. He explained that he had a "fake" leg, and the other didn't work very well either. It wasn't the nicest prosthetic I had seen, but it got him around.

I drove Richie home to his little run-down shack up a hill off Fern Crescent. Fern Crescent is the gateway to the beautiful Golden Ears Provincial Park, so even though his house was a bit of a dump (for lack of a better word), the forested surroundings were pristine.

Believe it or not, I accepted Richie's invitation to go in. He gave me the grand tour of his two-roomed cabin in the woods like he was showing me a palace. The place was a mess and there was some guy sleeping on his couch. He told me he liked to help people out if they needed a place to stay. He told me he didn't have any electricity, but he happily made do with the wood-burning stove. He introduced me to his cat and he took me out on his "beautiful" back deck to observe the gorgeous view of the magnificent trees.

I quickly learned that Richie thought he was a rich man. But over time, I also learned he was very aware of his poverty.

In the Book of Matthew, the first book of the New Testament, Jesus delivers an excellent message, called "The Sermon on the Mount." It's found in chapters five through seven, and it's convicting, compelling, and beautiful. If you have never read it, it's a great read. If you have, but it's been a while—it might be just what you need right now.

Anyway, the sermon starts with the Beatitudes (which means "supreme blessedness" or "happiness"). The first Beatitude is, "Blessed are the poor in spirit, for theirs is the kingdom of heaven." While I understand other Beatitudes, such as, "Blessed are the merciful, for they will be shown mercy," and " Blessed are the peacemakers, for they will be called sons of God," this one about being "poor in spirit," I didn't really understand, and then came Richie to illustrate.

"The teaching of the Sermon on the Mount produces despair in the natural man—the very thing Jesus means it to do. As long as we have a self-righteous, conceited notion that we can carry out our Lord's teaching, God will allow us to go on until we break our ignorance over some obstacle, then we are willing to come to Him as paupers and receive from Him. 'Blessed are the paupers in spirit,' that is the first principle in the Kingdom of God."
Oswald Chambers

For the next ten years or so, I saw Richie on and off. I picked him up when I saw him hitchhiking; he sometimes drove by me in a run-down vehicle, waving and honking. I brought him to our house a couple of times and Mike and I went to his. I got to know Richie fairly well, although some things were never talked about. I suspected he had lots of troubles over the course of his lifetime. Perhaps there was mental illness, drug and/or alcohol abuse, or whatever, but the man at some point was reborn. He shared his grief about his mother's death and not seeing his children and ex-wife in years, and he shared his love for the Lord and had a light about him.

The last few times I saw Richie, he sang to me a song he had written. I wish I'd jotted down the words. He had sung to me before, hymns mostly—he had a very nice voice. But this song was special; it was his and he was happy to have someone listen. I can still see his toothless grin mouth the wonderful praises.

One day, Mike and I went to check in on Richie at his house, but it was all boarded up. A neighbour said we might find him at the hospital, and we did. He had heath issues, but was only there for a couple of days and then he went to stay with a friend in Coquitlam, a city about a half hour away. We went to pick him up one day to take him for dinner at our church and saw his new place was actually someone's garage.

The last time I talked to Richie was on the phone. He called to tell me something, but he was really hard to understand. I wondered if he had been drinking or if he was that way because of his illness; but after that, I never heard from him again. Mike and Richie's pastor from his church were in contact, trying to find Richie. Eventually, the Pastor called to say Richie had passed away. We attended his funeral along with a few parishioners. It was lovely and I know Richie would have liked it; we sang some old hymns.

"The New Testament notices things that do not seem worthy of notice by our standards. 'Blessed are the poor in spirit ...' This literally means, 'Blessed are the paupers.' Paupers are remarkably commonplace! The preaching of today tends to point out a person's strength of will or the beauty of his character—things that are easily noticed. At the foundation of Jesus Christ's kingdom is the genuine loveliness of those who are commonplace."
Oswald Chambers

Richie Rich was a rich poor man and my life is richer from knowing him.

Richer Than You Think—December 5, 2013

The more things we lose because of ALS, the richer we become ... does that make any sense? Perhaps this "devastating" illness isn't as devastating as we thought. Almost everything about our lives has changed, but the best things remain. Mike has lost his job, his home, most possessions, the ability to drive, write, run, walk, talk, eat, and so on. But the best things in Mike's life still belong to him, such as love, laughter, family, friends ... we are richer than we think.

"You're Richer Than You Think." That's a Scotiabank slogan. My mom worked for Scotiabank as a teller most of her working years and loved it and they loved her ... she was their best employee! Anyway, I wonder if those Scotiabank advertising geniuses know how insightful their "You're richer than you think" slogan really is. Apart from high-interest savings accounts, investment plans, mutual funds, and RRSPs, their "You're richer than you think" is very true for most of us.

The other night, my parents, Mike's mum, his sisters, Aileen and Pat, and Mike and I watched some old home movies. One video we watched was one Mike and I made for my mom for her sixtieth birthday (sixteen years ago). There were some skits Mike did with my mom, and a song-and-dance routine he and our children did together to the song "Sixteen Candles." They just changed it a little and sang "Sixty Candles" instead; the cake was pretty much on fire with that many lit candles. It was one of those "you had to be there" things, so I'm not going to try to describe it. It was funny, though. Super funny! We laughed and laughed. Being with family, laughing together, talking, sharing, and reminiscing; this is what it means to be "rich" and we are indeed richer than we think.

Travelling to Malawi, Africa on a few occasions has been an invaluable experience for all of us, especially for our kids. After observing how people live in this very poor country, they realized quickly that they are richer than they think.

Temperatures Rising—December 10, 2013

It's been really cold here this past week. I know compared to the rest of Canada it's almost tropical, but for us West Coasters, it's freezing. The temperature has been as low as minus eight degrees Celsius with the wind chill factor making it minus fifteen. Compared to Calgary (-28°) and other places across the country (-40°), it's pretty balmy here in the Vancouver area, but I'm a big baby and it's been way too cold for me!

Lying in bed the other morning, a little chilly and not quite awake yet, I was either dreaming or recalling a favourite memory in my slumberous state. Mike and I were in our old little room, in our old cozy bed all cuddled up together. He had his big strong arm around me pulling me up against his hot body. All tucked inside him, I felt warm and secure. Hidden under the covers, like two spoons in a dark drawer fitting perfectly together, quiet, and still on a cold winter's morning.

When fully awake, I decided that this is definitely what I miss the most.

Trying to describe that feeling of being enveloped in a warm body, being held and hugged … snow falling, temperature rising on a cold winter's morning; there aren't words to describe that feeling. I didn't realize at the time how wonderful, how exceptional it is to be held like that. But now I know and it's what I miss the most.

This morning, again feeling a little chilly and still sleepy, I decided to recreate the scene in reverse. With our beds pushed together, I rearranged Mike's pillows and nuzzled in next to him. My strong arm around his frailty, gently pulling my cool self up against his hot body. Hidden under the covers, not as perfect a fit, but still like two spoons in a dark drawer, quiet and still … snow falling, temperature rising on a cold winter's morning.

How wonderful, how exceptional it is to hold and be held like this!

Peace On Earth—December 29, 2013

This Christmas I was so excited about some of the gifts I gave. It's such a great feeling to find something special, for someone special, knowing the gift will mean a lot regardless of the size or cost. I was actually quite proud of myself and all my great finds. I thought for sure this year I was going to give more than I could ever receive … wrong!

My receiving started well before the twenty-fifth. One morning, Adele gave me some excuse why she had to leave my class early and then came back a few minutes later dressed as Mrs. Claus and accompanied by Santa. They presented me with a huge gift from friends in the fitness community. Fellow fitness instructors and many participants went in on the most amazing gift for me and Mike … I'm still in shock. Over seventy names were written on the cards that accompanied the gift. Wow!

I received many other special gifts as well, including one from Mike. With help from some elves (who happen to look a lot like his sisters), Mike gave me a gift that took my breath away. I will cherish his gift for the rest of my life. But as I ponder gifts given and received throughout the season, I continually give thanks for the best gift I was given ... another Christmas with Mike!

Every day with Mike is a gift and the peace we have in the midst of ALS is also an amazing gift. For Christians, Christmas is about the perfect gift given to an imperfect humanity on the very first Christmas: Jesus Christ. And the peace that comes from knowing Him is inconceivable.

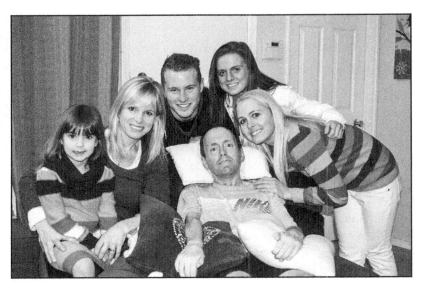

Leah, Nadine, Nathan, Madison, Erin, and Mike
Family photo by Ashley Wadhwani

I am not offended if you don't celebrate Christ at Christmas ... Season's Greetings and Happy Holidays to you for sure. But if you do celebrate Christ at Christmas and if you know Him personally every day of the year, then you may know about this peace that surpasses all understanding which I am talking about.

Oswald Chambers puts it this way: "When you really see Jesus, I defy you to doubt Him. If you see Him when He says, 'Let not your heart be troubled ...,' I defy you to worry. It is virtually impossible to doubt when He is there. Every time you are in personal contact with Jesus, His words are real to you. 'My peace I give you'—a peace which brings an unconstrained confidence and covers you completely, from the top of your head to the soles of your feet. 'Your life is hidden with Christ in God,' and the peace of Jesus Christ that cannot be disturbed has been imparted to you."

Peace on earth came in the form of a baby born in a manger; fully man, fully God ... the Messiah. Born to us ... a Saviour!

Merry Christmas, Season's Greetings, Happy Holidays ... Peace!

~ ~ ~ ~ ~ ~ ~

My fitness friends have blessed me over the years with many gifts and they continue to bless us and encourage us with their kindness and generosity.

Mike's gift to me was a beautiful silver jewellery box with a picture of the two of us on the front. Inside was a ring with my birthstone and engraved on the inside of the box were the words, "Double that and you got me."

Here's Hoping—January 10, 2014

The other day when I woke up, I lay in bed for a little while. I didn't feel like getting up. I could see through the slats of the blinds that it was still dark and I could hear the rain. Suddenly, I had Seasonal Affective Disorder (SAD) or at least I figured this is what it must feel like.

I talked myself into getting up, even though I didn't really have a choice. Mike and I have certain routines on certain days and on this day and three other days of the week I get him up early to accomplish certain tasks before the home care nurse comes. I can't roll over and go back to sleep … it's not an option. So I had to ignore feeling blue and begin the day.

When Mike and I finished our routine and the home care nurse took over, I was sure I could hear my bed calling me back. As tempting as it was to return to my cozy little hiding place, and regardless of how tired and unmotivated I felt, I resisted. I almost never go back to bed—I'm just not a good napper. I went for a walk instead. I needed to go to the store for something anyway, so on with the rubber boots and out with the umbrella and off I went. On a dry day, walking to the store or anywhere isn't unusual for me, but on a rainy day, I normally drive. Feeling lacklustre, I figured some fresh air would do the trick.

I started off pretty slow, but still went the long way. I realized I was going to need a lot of time to shake those blahs. I prayed and pondered and praised the Lord with a little bit of singing. By the time I got to the store, I was feeling a lot better.

I took an even longer route home and enjoyed walking through some neighbourhoods Mike and I have enjoyed walking through so many times together. I was glad I brought an umbrella, because it just rained harder, but that didn't bother me at all. I quite liked the rain … it made me hopeful for sunshine. I started to think about hope and the more I thought about it, the more hopeful I became. The more hopeful I became, the more skip in my step and my posture improved. I got wet on the final stretch home though … I put my umbrella down because it was blocking out the little bit of sunlight breaking through the clouds.

I don't know where my hope was when I woke up that morning, but it's back. That was Tuesday. The next day and the next day and the one after that—same darkness, same rain, but lots of hope!

Since Mike's ALS diagnosis almost three years ago, we have clung to hope ... we stick to it like glue! Whether it's a cure for the disease, a miracle for Mike and Neil and others with it, or whether it's another Christmas together or springtime ... we have hope and we aren't letting go!

I love *Merriam-Webster's* definition of hope: "To cherish a desire with anticipation and to expect with confidence." With hope anything can happen ... or at least something can happen. Without hope, dismay. Hope is a reason to get up in the morning ... hope is a rope ... hope trumps impossible!

Happy New Year, everyone! Here's to a year filled with HOPE!

A superman, the late Christopher Reeve said, "Once you choose hope, anything's possible."

Hidden Treasure—January 22, 2014

Maple Ridge is a fairly small town and it seems everywhere I go I bump into someone I know who asks me about Mike. It is nice so many people care, but I never really know what to say. I usually say he is well, but that can be a little confusing sometimes. For example, while Christmas shopping at Target last month, I bumped into a fellow soccer mom from years ago. She was pleasantly surprised when I answered her question, "How's Mike?" with "He's great!"

She assumed his illness wasn't progressing. I had to explain that his illness is progressing; but he is really good ... on the inside.

It's more than the positive attitude I have written about so many times. He is the same "Mike" inside ... funny, cheeky, silly, happy, smart! Even more than ever, because he has all this time to focus inward, unable to focus or dwell on his outside, like people have a tendency to do. He has had time to think about what is important and what isn't. He has contemplated life ... and death. There is prayer, reflection, and examination going on inside. While the outside is weak and frail, things on the inside have been shaped, sharpened, and shined ... I think of it as hidden treasure.

There is a chest of treasure inside him and I get excited when it's opened. On a regular basis, communication is simple in one way and often challenging in another way for Mike and me and anyone interacting with him. He will look to his right toward the thermostat if he wants the heat on or off. He looks further to the right, over his shoulder, if he wants his laptop. He will open his mouth slightly and look to his left if he needs suction. Saying "P" and looking toward the bathroom of course means he needs to go pee. I can understand quite a bit by the look in his eyes, the lifting of his eyebrows, a certain nod or motion of his head, and of course a big smile. We usually get by this way and it's good.

But what I love is when that treasure chest is opened and the wonderful world that exists in him is revealed. For instance, a while ago, Mike had a reaction to a new medication that kept him awake all night (several nights). We were both exhausted and frustrated, because he was so itchy and I, the scratcher, was unable to keep up with the itch and unable to understand where to scratch next. He was also restless and uncomfortable, and trying to tell me what he wanted was gruelling … for both of us. I was so mad at myself for not knowing what to do.

The next day, I had a Facebook message from Mike quoting George Costanza from Seinfeld. It said, "It's not you, it's me!" I laughed and cried. When he writes me a note on his computer or sends me a Facebook message, I think, "There he is … there's my Mike."

I love hearing from him. He sends me messages to explain any earlier miscommunication. He'll write, "What I was trying to tell you before …" I had a message a few weeks ago from him relaying details of a dream he had. I'll be out and I'll get a message from him with his numbers for a Sports Action ticket. He messages me to tell me I'm doing a good job, that the insurance is due on the van, and what he thinks we should give a dear friend in need for her birthday.

His post, "Ahoy, Matey" reveals to us that treasure inside I speak of. The story contains historical information, education, wit, and a few corny jokes that he has told a few times before … it's Mike! I loved that story then and I love it now.

Mike has a new communication device called a DynaVox. He uses the head mouse he has been using on his laptop to control the cursor and it's completely hands-free. There is a keyboard of the alphabet and a variety of common words to choose from to spell out whatever he wants to say. He can hit a "speak" key and the device will speak out loud what he has written.

On the weekend, with a group of us here celebrating Mike's "birthday week," we had a great time listening to Mike. He had us all in stitches. Leah, who is four now, was especially amused.

She hasn't really had any conversation with Mike. She was surprised and a little shocked to hear from him.

Mike was telling Leah to put the crickets she had in the turtle aquarium; she and her dad bought the crickets for her frog to eat, but she wanted to keep them as pets instead. Mike was telling her that, "Turtles like to play with crickets; they ride them on their backs." She got a real kick out of that!

"Therefore, we do not lose heart. Though outwardly we are wasting away, yet inwardly we are being renewed day by day. For our light and momentary troubles are achieving for us an eternal glory that far outweighs them all. So we fix our eyes not on what is seen, but on what is unseen. For what is seen is temporary but what is unseen is eternal."
II Corinthians 4:16-18

P.S. In Mike's blog post, "Hawaii Five Old," written two years ago, he tells about his achievement of reaching the age of fifty. He said that anything beyond fifty was icing on the cake. So I guess the last two years has all been icing. What a great way to look at life ... pretty sweet! His closing statement is: "We can't regret growing old as it is a privilege that many people do not experience." Happy Birthday also to our friend Neil (January 15) who is also battling ALS with courage, hope, and humour ... thanks for the laughs, buddy ... keep up the good work and the great jokes!

Till Death Do Us Part—January 28, 2014

I have really gotten used to living this way; that is with ALS. I kind of forget what normal is. This is normal now. Sometimes

I remember that ALS is going to steal Mike's every last breath and take his life, although I'm still not totally buying it. I can't see it; I don't believe it … most of the time.

I can't imagine my life without Mike. I'm not ready to let him go today, but I pray that when the time comes, I will be ready. I'll send him off with my blessing and I'll watch him fly away. It almost sounds romantic when I put it like that, but it will be tragic. Sorrow also comes to mind, but so does joy, and when it's time there will be that as well. I know because the two, sorrow and joy, have commingled in my life since Mike's diagnosis and it's the joy that has been my strength.

> *"[F]or the joy of the Lord is your strength."*
> **Nehemiah 8:10**

I was just a girl when I said, "I do." I took Mike and he took me for better or worse, for richer or poorer, in sickness and in health, till death do us part. I didn't really know what that all meant when I agreed to it twenty-five years, seven months, and four days ago, but I do know what it means now. The last bit though, the part about "parting," that's a little hard to understand. Mike and I are one, like a piece of fabric; threads woven together. How does that just part? Is it like a ripping, a tearing, a cutting? Sounds painful! I know it will be. It already is. But the joy of having him in my life all these years will remain … and so will the love.

Sometimes I wonder where we would be without ALS, and believe it or not, I question if I'd go back. Don't get me wrong. Of course, I wouldn't wish ALS on my husband or on anyone. But what we have learned is invaluable and what we have overcome and what we have achieved is incredible and how we have experienced God and the joy that comes from knowing Him, trusting Him, and abiding in Him is indescribable ... I wouldn't trade all that for anything. What is also indescribable is the love; God's love, the love of family and friends, and our love for each other ... that doesn't part when we do; that lasts forever!

My sleeves are covered in tears as I write this and I wonder if it's too sad to share, but it's part of our "normal" lives with ALS, so here it is. I hope it will inspire all to appreciate every minute, to look to the Lord and experience His joy, which brings strength, and to cherish the love.

> *"It happens every time you praise God. It is instantly felt in His presence. This joy comes from a source that never runs dry. It becomes your strength. No matter what else is happening it's that underlying feeling that everything is going to ultimately be good."*
> **Stormie Omartian**

Hold On and Let Go—February 11, 2014

Last week when I was driving Mike to his bath appointment, I looked at him through the rearview mirror and observed the content look on his face. I kept alternating my gaze between his face in the mirror and the road in front of me through the windshield. I couldn't help but smile and think how well he rolls with the punches.

People say what a difficult time we must be going through, but I don't feel like that at all. It's been difficult at times, but not necessarily a difficult time. It's been a time to grow and to learn.

It's been a time to put things in proper perspective. It's a process for sure, but we are learning to hold on and let go. We let go of things in our lives that hinder and distract us like worry and fear; and we hold on to things that enhance and beautify our lives like faith, hope, love, and all the other wonderful outpourings of the Lord.

Good things come from bad things all the time. That's how God works. He redeems things. God has done it with ALS in our lives a lot. I am constantly reminded of the popular Bible verse, Romans 8:28, which says, "And we know that in all things God works for the good of those who love Him, who have been called according to His purpose."

We all have trials in our lives … we all have troubles … some more than others. What I have learned is that the trials in life accelerate growth and learning. And without adversity you never really grow … adversity is a "good" thing. For us with ALS, it's been an opportunity to not only grow more, but to know more, to love more, to give and forgive more, and to live life to the fullest.

"We have to keep letting go, and slowly and surely the great full life of God will invade us in every part, and men will take knowledge of us that we have been with Jesus."
Oswald Chambers

Faced With Grace—February 27, 2014

I come face to face with God's grace every day and even more so every night. It's rare for me and Mike to have an uninterrupted night of sleep. I can't remember the last time it happened. Some nights we are awake two or three times and some nights we are awake every hour or more. I sleep lightly, like a mother of a newborn baby … on guard and ready to meet any need of the helpless little love of her life. But for over three years, my delight in responding to Mike's needs in the middle of the night has diminished.

When Mike needs something in the wee hours of the morning, it's a bit of a guessing game. Maybe he needs the head of his bed raised or lowered, or maybe he needs something scratched, or maybe he needs to turn over, or maybe he needs to go pee. To find out what Mike needs, I have to turn the light on, because I have to see his face to communicate with him. Even his nods lately are somewhat hard to read … was that a "yes" or a "no"? His eyes tell me the most. I run through a series of questions; sometimes I get it right away and sometimes it takes a while, and every time, Mike is patient with me. However, my patience wears thin after the second or third wakeup call.

When I get up to attend to Mike, I put on a sweater, socks, and sometimes shoes, so I can get a grip on the laminate floor if he wants to turn over. Waking up is one thing, but having to get up and dressed is another. Getting out of my warm, cozy bed is usually the last thing I want to do and this is where I come face to face with God's grace. Sometimes I'm a little disoriented, sometimes I get frustrated, even angry almost. Not at Mike, but at the situation, not even at the situation; I guess it's sleep deprivation. I don't say anything in my displeasure, I keep it inside. I'm sure Mike can tell though, because I'm not cheerful like I am in the day. Perhaps that's normal, but I don't want to be normal. I want to serve my husband with a happy heart all the time, sleep deprived or totally rested.

God is using this experience in my life in a couple of ways.

One of which is to show me another side of His grace. God is with me in the middle of the night, in the darkness just before I turn on the light. By His grace, I get up once more to serve my beloved husband. God enables me. He carries me. He loves me. When I think I can't do it again, He says, "Yes, you can! I am here and I will help you." And He does.

God is also using this experience in my life to teach me about surrender. It's easy to say, "I surrender all" to God, but is it easy to do? Jesus said in order to follow Him you have to deny yourself (Luke 9:23). Wow, that's a little beyond me. But by God's grace, He helps me make strides in that direction and in the middle of the night, I am humbled and grateful every time He says, "Yes, you can!"

ALS has forced Mike to surrender everything. He hasn't had a choice in surrendering, but he has had a choice in how he surrenders. He has done it with such dignity.

ALS has forced me to surrender a lot as well and God continues to call me to surrender it all. And He has given me an excellent role model: Mike!

I can't guarantee that lack of sleep won't get the best of me, but I can guarantee that God's grace will ... it has!

"Once we are totally surrendered to God, He will work through us all the time."
Oswald Chambers

Every Minute Matters—March 8, 2014

Ahh, the sounds of an NHL Hockey game ... the cheering of happy fans, the familiar voices of enthusiastic commentators, and the signature organ music ... it's all music to Mike's ears.

The National Hockey League took a three-week time-out for the Winter Olympics and Mike is glad the NHL is back in full swing, even though he really enjoyed watching the Olympics.

We had the Olympic games on almost all day every day. It was exciting, it was exhilarating, and it was a little nerve-racking. It's so much more than sporting events and the world's finest athleticism—it's incredible stories of determination, self-sacrifice, and teamwork. We were brought to tears many times witnessing perfect performances, record-breaking feats, devastating mistakes, wins, losses, and extraordinary comebacks.

We will never forget the women's gold medal hockey game between Canada and the US. Talk about a "comeback"! Mike says it was one of the greatest comebacks in hockey history.

The Canadian women were down two nothing with less than four minutes to go in the third period. Both teams were playing brilliantly and the Americans surely thinking they'd got this one, when Canada scores with only three minutes and twenty seconds left in the game. And then they score again with only fifty-five seconds left in the game. And then they score in overtime to win the game and take the gold!

It was a lesson for all of us … never give up! It was a great reminder … it's not over until it's over! It was a profound statement … every minute counts! It's quite like how we started thinking when Mike was diagnosed with a terminal illness.

A few of the Canadian women left a note on the men's locker room door before the men's semi-final game against the US. In part it said, "Tonight is yours. Own the moment. We are proof that every minute matters … Earn every inch, dictate the pace and go get 'em!"

The men won that semi-final game 1-0 and went on to win the gold medal game against Sweden, 3-0. Wow, that's great, but back to the women—how excellent of them to educate us on what a difference five minutes can make. They didn't give up. They knew "it's not over until it's over" and they finished extremely well … every minute matters indeed!

It reminds me of a friend of mine—a friend who finished well. On a number of occasions throughout the course of our friendship, she had kindly declined any invitation to hear about my faith and the Lord I worship and follow.

A week before she died, even though very ill, she still wasn't really interested in talking about God or being prayed for. But only a few days after that, conscious but unresponsive, lying in her hospital bed waiting to escape her sickly body, she had a change of heart.

I sat beside her and took her hand in mine. Before I said anything about God, I told her what a good wife and outstanding mother she was. I told her what a beautiful person she was inside and out. And I told her what a wonderful friend she was and how she'd enriched my life.

Then I simply told her about God's incredible love for her. How Jesus was waiting for her with open arms. How she could—right there and then—open the door and invite Him in … accepting Him as her Lord and Saviour. I said a prayer and told her she could pray along with me in her heart to receive forgiveness of sin and peace.

When I finished, she rubbed her thumb on the top of my hand and said, "Thank you so much for coming, Nadine."

We spent the rest of our visit basking in God's goodness and a couple of days later she went to be with Him. She fought hard, she finished well, and every minute mattered!

Yesterday (March 7) marked the third anniversary of Mike's diagnosis. I am so proud of him. Still content and still so brave, he is finishing well; but it isn't over until it's over. Every minute definitely matters, and we give thanks for each one of them.

"However, I consider my life worth nothing to me; my only aim is to finish the race and complete the task the Lord Jesus has given me—the task of testifying to the gospel of God's grace."
Acts 20:24

P.S. Madison and Hayley Wickenheiser played in the same hockey league last year - the Canadian Interuniversity Sport league. Because it wasn't an Olympic year, Wickenheiser was playing for the University of Calgary and Madison plays at the neighbouring university, Mount Royal. Wickenheiser is considered the best female hockey player of all time. She has won four Olympic gold medals and one silver. What a great opportunity for Madison to check Hayley ... and she kept her from scoring any goals!

Madison has since made the very difficult decision to leave her hockey scholarship and a team and coaches she loves, and move back home to be with her family and spend what time is left with her dad. She played hockey this season on a local team, with her old coaches and some long-time friends. She plans to go back to school next year and take a program offered here at a local college.

~ ~ ~ ~ ~ ~ ~

We come into this world with nothing and we leave with nothing, and it doesn't really matter what we have and what we accumulate in between, because most of us, like Richie Rich, eventually realize, we are poor.

"The bedrock in Jesus Christ's kingdom is poverty, not possession; not decisions for Jesus Christ, but a sense of absolute futility—I cannot begin to do it. Then Jesus says, Blessed are you. That is the entrance, and it does take us a long while to believe we are poor! 'Blessed are you, because it is through your poverty that you can enter My kingdom.' I cannot enter His kingdom by virtue of my goodness—I can only enter it as an absolute pauper."
Oswald Chambers

Chapter 16
You Can Kiss Me Now

This illness gets really tough. I blog about the highs and lows—the good, the bad, the ugly, but I barely touch the surface of it. The emotional toll is huge and the physical toll on both of us is obviously enormous. Every time I get to the end of myself, I remind myself that Mike is the one with the illness—I can walk and talk and breathe easily. I have to pick myself up and try to keep going because he does ... he's better than me.

Mike and I were interviewed for a short film about ALS and the ALS Society of BC. The young filmmaker, Tyler had an uncle who'd died of ALS and Tyler wanted to promote the ALS Society, highlighting what they do and what they offer to those with the illness and their families, in the hopes to raise money for it. During the interview, using Mike's DynaVox, Mike said to the interviewer that my life is on hold while I take care of him, and then he broke down. I broke down too, because I was sad to know Mike thought that—I don't think that. I quickly said with tears that my life was not on hold; I said that this was just my life right now ... our lives for now ... we are in it together and I cherish every minute, because when it's over, we're apart.

I'll never forget the time I drove Carol's son to the pharmacy to get his daily dose of methadone. He talked a little bit about his drug addiction and shared some grief with me. He told me that he just wanted his life back. Since then, I always pray, "May he soon have his life back." Young, smart, talented, funny, charismatic, dramatic, handsome ... I ask that he get his life back!

Mike and I don't ask for our lives back anymore. We accept this life now with ALS. We just pray that God continues to give us strength every day and we cherish every minute still left together.

This was yesterday, August 29, 2014 ... this is how tough it is some days ...

Mike needed an enema, because the one he had the day before didn't produce the results he was hoping for and he was feeling uncomfortable. We were going to do it first thing in the morning like we normally do four days a week, but the community Occupational Therapist wanted to come in and observe how the home support worker transfers him out of bed, to the shower chair, to the shower, etc., because Mike's care plan needed updating (which was way overdue) and the thought was that perhaps Mike needed a second support worker (which is way overdue as well).

So just before noon, when I went in to see if Mike wanted a tube feed, he asked me to give him an enema. I'm still the only one who gives him enemas. The home care worker was still here, but she isn't allowed to help me (it's a Workers' Compensation Board (WCB) of BC Insurance thing). So, using the lifts like always now, I transferred Mike to his commode and took him to the bedroom where I transferred him to the bed (with the head of the bed in an upright position). I had a little bit of assistance from the home care person … she handed me things I needed. After I got Mike in his bed, I lowered the head of the bed so I could turn him on his side. After lowering his head, I proceeded to start to roll him and he started to choke (this is common when he lies flat), so I quickly got him back on his back and elevated the head of the bed again. After he cleared his throat, I tried again. After trying three times with the same result, we gave up, and I got him back up, transferred him to his commode, and took him back to his chair and transferred him there and got him comfortable. This process is very tiring for both of us.

Later in the afternoon, after watching *Judge Judy*, we tried again (the home care person was long gone). This time Mike didn't choke, we did the enema, and I got him to the bathroom. Mike spent a lot of time there, but again, not the result he was hoping for, so back to the drawing board … we did another enema. Meanwhile, the faucet was turned on in his mouth and I couldn't keep up with suctioning the stream of saliva. Mike is on a new medication to help dry up secretions and it has made a difference, but not yesterday … it was back to the constant flow. And his poor head kept falling forward as he tried to deal with the pooling in his mouth.

Thankfully, the second enema was successful. My back was breaking and my head was aching and Mike might have had whiplash, but he was smiling, so we were both happy. I gave him a tube feed in there somewhere and his meds a little later and kept suctioning, and by the time we were done it was 10:00 p.m. (we started at 5:00 p.m.). I was relieved it was bedtime, but Mike continued to try to clear his throat for about another half hour. He stayed on his commode and I kept doing everything I could to help him. Then he had to go pee ... with urgency! I ran to get his urinal and as I ran back I could hear the pee hitting the laminate floor and I yelled, "Nooooo!" I hadn't returned the bucket to the commode after cleaning it.

While on my hands and knees, I wiped up the pee and sobbed. That was it ... I just cried my eyes out, while Mike sat slumped in his chair, saliva running down and off his chin soaking his shirt. It was like I just couldn't take it anymore. I was so exhausted, but far more upsetting than my small exhaustion problem, was Mike's enormous problem—this stupid ALS. Sometimes I can't believe he lives like this!

But that was yesterday and today is today and God's mercies are new every morning.

While we don't ask for our old lives back any more, we often long for our new lives. In Brady Toops' rendition of "Swing Low Sweet Chariot," he sings, "No more worry, no more pain, every doubt erased. No more troubles weighing down my soul, comin' for to carry me home."

"Yet what we suffer now is nothing compared to the glory He will reveal to us later."
Romans 8:18, NLT

You Can Kiss Me Now—March 15, 2014

I wouldn't trade the last three years with ALS for anything. I know that sounds a little crazy, but let me explain. Some women and men lose their husbands, their wives suddenly. There is no warning. Like my friend's friend who lost her husband in a work-related accident. She got an unexpected call one day … just like that … he was gone. I wonder what their last words were. Did they kiss before he left for work that day? Or was he scrambling to get out the door while she scrambled eggs, packed lunches, and got the kids up and ready for school? Because that's how it is … that's what life is like.

Pre-ALS, Mike and I were often going in different directions— we were like two ships passing in the night, literally, because Mike worked full-time nights as well as some days and afternoons. We didn't always kiss hello and goodbye, and our "I love Yous" were few and far between.

But one day, someone wearing a white jacket holding a clipboard and a bunch of test results said to me, "You have three to five years to tell your husband how much you love him." I got a warning. My friend's friend didn't. No one told her the morning of her husband's death that she had three to five hours to tell him how much she loved him. No one told her to make sure she kissed him goodbye that day before he left.

At first I thought the doctor in the white coat with the bad news was our enemy, but now I believe she was a friend, a messenger of good news. I was given three to five years to kiss Mike every morning, every night, and every time I go out and come back again. I got a warning. My friend's friend didn't get a warning and my guess is she would tell me I'm really lucky.

One day a few weeks ago, I was scrambling to get out the door. I can't remember if I was going to teach a class or if I had an appointment, but wherever I was going I was running a little late. I was gathering everything I needed for my time out and I was making sure Mike was all ready for his time with his caregiver. I always make sure Mike is comfortable before I walk away and on this particular day, it took a little longer to get everything just right. Mike watched me buzz around like a bee and then just when I was ready, I could see he had something to tell me. I was hoping we could make it quick and sure enough he softly spelled it out with ease: "y-o-u c-a-n k-i-s-s m-e n-o-w."

Wow, I almost forgot. I almost forgot the most important part of my leaving. It reminds me of when I was a little girl and my grandpa would say when we were about to part, "You forgot something." I would kiss his cheek and he would kiss mine. It's a memory forever etched in my mind.

So ALS I guess, could be considered a gift. I know I might not feel that way every day, but today I give thanks for ALS. This is the first time I have given thanks for this debilitating disease. Mike gave thanks for ALS shortly after he was diagnosed. I'll never forget when he said thank you to God for the things he wanted and the things he didn't want in his life like ALS. He trusted God knew what He was doing.

"Rejoice always, pray continually, give thanks in all circumstances; for this is God's will for you in Christ Jesus."
I Thessalonians 5:16-18

Our love would never have known these depths had Mike been taken away suddenly. Instead, we were given three to five years to rejoice, pray, and give thanks together every day. And I wouldn't trade it for anything!

~ ~ ~ ~ ~ ~ ~

My Auntie Marguerite lost her true love suddenly. My uncle Trevor went out one day to fly his plane and didn't come back again. I'm the same age as her oldest son, Sean—we were ten when this tragedy happened.

I will never forget the afternoon I spent years ago with my Aunty Marguerite reminiscing about the love of her life. We laughed so hard and cried a lot too as she relayed some hilarious stories of their on-again, off-again courtship. Despite their bumpy start, they were destined to be together and got married at a young age. She read me some of the love letters he wrote her. There was so much sorrow and so much joy in those treasured notes and in my aunt's voice as she read them to me. I was sad for her and happy for her at the same time; her beloved wasn't there with her, but it was like he wasn't gone. Their young love was suspended in time but life had moved on.

Shortly after Mike's diagnosis, Sean messaged me and shared a little bit about how painful it was to lose his dad suddenly and at such a young age, and how it is still so difficult. He told me to tell my kids to soak up every moment they can with their dad. "Make a point of remembering things. Find out what he's about, where he's been, and where he came from. Record his voice, take video, all that stuff (we never had it back then)."

Sean is an excellent dad. Perhaps losing his daddy at age ten has caused him to cherish parenthood more than the average person. Maybe he doesn't take one minute as "dad" and one precious moment with his children for granted.

My blog post, "You Can Kiss Me Now," changed my life. I

remember completing this post and feeling free. I remember giving thanks for ALS and feeling like a weight had been lifted off me. I became more grateful than ever for the time we have together.

Sunny—March 26, 2014

The sun was shining in our bedroom this morning well before I opened the blinds. Mike woke up with a smile on his face that wouldn't quit. He always smiles when he first sees me, but this one didn't stop … it was like he had a secret or something.

Since writing my recent blog post "Faced With Grace," in which I talk about living with a lack of sleep, we have slept! It's been great to get a full night's sleep … with only one or two interruptions. Mike has been more comfortable and able to sleep well, so I sleep well and we both feel better. That might explain the constant smile this morning or Mike *does* have a secret. Nevertheless, it was the perfect way to start the day.

Perfect Timing—April 6, 2014

Madison just turned twenty. When I told my sister I was a little sad that I didn't have any more teenagers, she looked at me like I was crazy and my niece Michaela said, "Aunty, you still have me and Luke." Michaela just turned fourteen and Luke will be thirteen in a couple of days. That was sweet and it made me feel better for sure.

Even though Madison is all grown up, I still give her lots of unsolicited advice. "Madison, make sure you lock your truck."

"Madison, don't leave your bank card lying around."

"Madison, call me when you get there."

"Madison, rinse that dish, clean that up, put that away, do this, don't do that."

I'm really not a bossy person, but poor Madison, who is a little too relaxed for my liking, and somewhat disorganized, gets an earful from me every other day. I am the youngest child as well, so I can relate ... a little.

When Mike was diagnosed with ALS, we gave thanks that our children were grown—Erin was twenty-two, Nathan was twenty, and Madison was seventeen. The day Mike was diagnosed, Erin and Nathan went and picked Madison up from school so they could gently break the bad news to their little sister. I really appreciated it and I'm sure their bond grew stronger that day.

As timing goes ... to be given this diagnosis ... it wasn't bad. There definitely isn't a good time to be diagnosed with a terminal illness, but the timing could have been worse. Our children were at the age when they knew their dad well and had already made a million memories with him. And Mike thought if he could see his kids well into their twenties, that would be pretty great.

I just finished reading a book called *Heavy*. It's about a young family's first year with ALS. Todd Neva, who was diagnosed in June 2010, tells their story from his perspective with journal entries at the end of each chapter by Kristin Neva, his wife. I really liked the two perspectives. The book was well written and easy to read.

Unlike ours, Todd and Kristin's children were small when Todd was diagnosed with ALS. Their daughter was four and their son was just a baby. This would definitely add to the grief ... I can't imagine! Our children were raised, but Kristin would have to take care of her husband and her children, and will most likely (if this illness takes the same course it has in most cases) be a single young mom … eventually.

Todd writes about the sadness of not walking his daughter down the aisle on her wedding day or teaching her how to change the oil in her car. He worries that his son won't remember much about him. That is tough for sure. Todd and Kristin have a strong faith in God so, as difficult as it is, I'm sure they trust God's timing.

In our case, Mike may not escort his daughters down the aisle on their wedding days either, but he has been to all his children's graduations and many other special events. He has been to Erin's classroom where she works as a teacher. He has watched Nathan become a dad and do an excellent job raising his daughter so far. And he has seen Madison reach her twenties and become a fine young adult like her sister and brother.

Mike thinks of it as good timing. His kids (and granddaughter) are the pride of his life and he considers himself extremely blessed to have watched his children grow into kind, compassionate, caring, productive, outstanding adults.

Nathan took Erin out to her car the other day when they were here, so he could show her where the oil goes and give her other pointers under the hood. That brought Mike comfort and was a reminder to him that our children have each other. They help and support one another and always will.

I'm sure this thought brings Todd Neva comfort too. His children have each other and will surely help and support one another as they grow and live the rest of their lives. I'm sure his children, like our children, will also help each other keep memories of their dad alive and fresh in their minds. You hear our children often say, "Remember when Dad did this or that?" Laughter usually accompanies their reminiscing ... which puts a smile on Mike's face every time.

If you have given the throne of your life to God, if you trust Him and believe He knows what's best and does what's best, then you have to believe His timing is right—that His timing is perfect.

In my Amazon book review of *Heavy*, I said, "*Heavy* has made me feel a little lighter." I could relate to so much of Neva's story and somehow that is encouraging.

The following is part of Kristin's journal entry in Chapter 16 from February 2010:

"I asked my counsellor if he thought it is true that God doesn't give us more than we can handle.

"'I think that God always gives us more than we can handle,' he said. 'Life's unfair and unkind at times. The question is how do we muddle through?'

"Since Todd's diagnosis, I have been struggling to comprehend why God is allowing this in our lives, and why there is so much suffering in the world. In John 9, in the story of Jesus and the blind man, the disciples ask Jesus, 'Who sinned, this man or his parents, that he was born blind?'

"'Neither,' Jesus replies, 'But this happened so that the work of God might be displayed in his life.'...

"I can't wrap my mind around God's sovereignty paired with the bad things that happen in life. But maybe I don't need to. Maybe the point of the story of the blind man is that God through His grace can redeem any situation, and even bring out of it purpose and meaning.

"'Do you think that God planned our ALS or do you think He allowed it to happen?' I asked Todd.

"'I don't know,' he replied. 'What I do know is that there is a right way to respond.'

"'Maybe we don't need to have it all figured out, rather, we need to trust that God is in control and is working in our lives. God gives us more than we can handle, but it is not more than He can handle.'"

The Great Exchange—April 17, 2014

Last week, Mike had his feeding tube changed. It had been over a year since the first feeding tube was put in. When we went in October to have the tube changed, the doctor told us it was still good for another few months. Because sedation is required, and because Mike is nervous to be sedated in his condition with ALS, he wanted to wait—he wasn't going to have the procedure any earlier than necessary.

We were assured that having the tube changed was quick and easy ... compared to the last procedure of having the tube placed for the first time, which was tough on Mike. We were in the hospital for a few days ... recovering in Mike's condition isn't easy.

Mike's parents and sisters Aileen and Pat were here for that first procedure and came back for the appointment last week (they come every two to three months for a visit anyway).

Remembering the physical toll the first procedure took on Mike and the emotional toll it took on the rest of us, we were all a little tense.

Sure enough, the procedure was pretty quick and easy. Because of Mike's excess saliva issue though, when the doctor sprayed his throat with a numbing spray he immediately started to cough (clear his throat) and continued for a few hours after, but other than that he was fine.

During the procedure, Mike's family waited patiently in the waiting area, and Elanna and I stood right outside the surgical room door. When it was over, I'm sure our collective sighs of relief could be heard throughout the ward. Mike recovered in the recovery area for a couple of hours with his family taking turns to see how he was doing, and then we were free to go home.

When we left, I wheeled Mike out to the waiting room where everyone rose to their feet and cheered. It was fitting to celebrate at a time like this. Mike had a big smile on his face and was so encouraged!

Speaking of celebration, this past Sunday was Palm Sunday. On Palm Sunday, Christians celebrate the triumphal entry of Jesus into Jerusalem one week before Easter. When Jesus rode into Jerusalem on a donkey, less than a week before his death by crucifixion, the celebratory crowd laid their cloaks on the road before him along with palm branches; some waved palm branches in the air.

> *"The next day the great crowd that had come for the festival heard that Jesus was on his way to Jerusalem. They took palm branches and went out to meet Him, shouting, 'Hosanna!' 'Blessed is He who comes in the name of the Lord!' 'Blessed is the King of Israel!'"*
> **John 12:12-13**

The Pastor at church titled his sermon, "The Entrance of a King" and delivered a good message. I'll admit though I didn't catch all of it, because I nodded off a few times (not because it was boring; I was just tired). I was wide-awake, however, at the end when the Pastor finished his sermon with a question. He said, "What do you need to let go of, so you can pick up a palm leaf and celebrate?"

Wow, he totally caught me off guard. I became a little emotional when I closed my eyes and saw myself with a heavy load that made it impossible to raise my palm. I thought I had let go, but apparently, I picked some cares back up again. I hadn't realized my praise was impaired by burdens.

Whether it's cares or worries or sin or regret or unforgiveness, it weighs us down and keeps us from raising our palms and praising Him.

At Easter or anytime, you can cast your cares at the foot of the cross and raise your palms and celebrate!

"Blessed is He who comes in the name of the Lord!"
John 12-13

Oh Crap!—May 9, 2014

Lately when people ask me how Mike is doing, I respond, "He's still smiling." I think my response says a lot. It says he is still happy and he is still able to move some facial muscles. The thing is Mike is almost completely paralyzed. The paralysis has been gradual over the last three years, but the changes in the last few months, although still subtle, have been the most impactful. I should clarify that this paralysis with ALS means he can't move, but he still has feeling. In fact, Mike can be very sensitive to touch.

The subtle changes of late are the hardest for me emotionally and physically. Emotionally, because it's the final stage of paralysis, and physically, because my caregiving has become more complicated.

Mike's dead weight makes it difficult for us to do the pivot transfers we have been doing for so long. I used to pull Mike up to standing and then brace him around his upper arms and move his feet with my feet inch by inch to get him from his chair to his wheelchair or commode to the bed and so on. Now, I mostly use the lifts. His arms and legs haven't worked for a long time, but his core muscles and neck muscles are failing as well causing him to lean a lot when sitting upright and his head to fall forward … or back. There is a lot of fidgeting and fussing, propping and pulling, shifting and shoving, but he keeps smiling.

Mike has had a lot of phlegm lately. Around about the time he had his feeding tube changed last month, we have been doing more suctioning … of phlegm and saliva. I go in to the back of his throat with the suction, using a flashlight to see my way. Poor guy—gagging as I wrestle with the glue-like substance. It's pretty gross, but I love clearing his throat, knowing it's got to feel good. I have referred to a few of the bigger clumps of stuff as "magic loogies" (a Seinfeld thing) and Mike keeps smiling.

Last week, Mike suffered with another type of congestion … if you know what I mean. Poor guy couldn't go. Four days in and his smile had dwindled. Mike is regular … we make sure of it. We have a routine—that, along with excellent nutrition, thankfully, Mike's pretty clear.

Mike always called a bowel movement a "TC," which stands for "Thomas Crapper." Mike said that Thomas Crapper was the inventor of the toilet, so it only made sense to call a "BM" a "TC." Mike had a lot of stories and you never knew which ones to believe. A little research tells me this story is partly true. Thomas Crapper didn't invent the flush toilet, but he did develop it and had some important related inventions.

If someone in our house wasn't feeling well, Mike would ask, "Have you had a TC?" If someone wasn't quite right, he'd say, "Go have a TC!" The kids got a kick out of it when they were little and eventually it was just part of our lingo.

Having a good TC can be difficult once in a while for anyone, but especially for someone who is sedentary, like Mike ... it's a real bummer! It's been an issue for Mike just a couple of times, but not near as severe as last week. We tried everything—it was our whole focus for seven days. Everyone was concerned. My parents were calling, Elanna was asking, and the kids were texting me, "Has he gone yet?"

It was a long week, but on Sunday morning when Mike finally had the TC we were all praying for, the clouds opened up and I'm sure the "Hallelujah Chorus" could be heard for miles.

Mike's smile came right back ... and he's been smiling ever since!

Still Standing—May 25, 2014

Although neither of Mike's home teams, the Vancouver Canucks and the Toronto Maple Leafs, made it to the NHL playoffs this year, Mike is faithfully watching. The Montreal Canadiens, (the only Canadian team to make it to the playoffs) are his favourite of course, but he was also cheering for the Columbus Blue Jackets, because the Jackets' young and talented Ryan Johansen from Port Moody, BC played on the same team as the young and talented Nathan Sands from Maple Ridge. They played

Major Midget Hockey together on the Vancouver North East Chiefs. Nathan still plays a little hockey recreationally.

Mike was also cheering for the Colorado Avalanche, of course. Even though one of our all-time favourite players, Joe Sakic, retired in 2009, I suppose we will always root for his team. The only other team Mike was cheering for that is still in the playoffs along with the Canadiens is the New York Rangers. We particularly like the Rangers this year because of the coach … the Canucks' former coach, Alain Vigneault.

Here we are already in the third round of the playoffs and it's Montreal versus New York … they are three games in. The first two games were disappointing to say the least. New York won both games: 7-2 and 3-1. The third game was a bit of a nailbiter, but Montreal scored early in overtime to win.

I never sit through a whole game. I do other things and just watch bits and pieces. If I can hear the crowd going wild, including Mike, I come and watch the replay. Highlights during intermission or at the end of the game get me all caught up and I pretty much know exactly what happened. Anyway, what I could tell from what I saw of that third game, New York was all over Montreal, but Montreal, two games down and fighting for their lives, did not give up! You gotta love that kind of determination!

It reminds me of Mike. I know I might sound like a broken record, but through every stage of this illness, he just doesn't give up! Unable to sit up straight with trunk muscles and neck muscles so much weaker now, he is still determined to stand every day … even for just a few minutes.

Sometimes it takes a while to get his feet right where he wants them. Once I get him up to a partial stand and prop him against his chair, I quickly get down and adjust his left foot (the weaker of the two). I put my shoulder against the outside of his left knee to stabilize his leg and then I adjust his foot with both my hands. With every little adjustment, I look up at his face to see if I've hit the sweet spot. He'll give me the eyebrows up signal (like thumbs up) to tell me "good." From there I prop pillows under his arms and quickly get the suction machine and suction his mouth. When first in that semi-standing position, before he is able to stretch himself to full standing, his head falls forward and all the saliva pools in the front of his mouth and slowly seeps through his lips. I sometimes feel a drop or two fall on my head, but first things first. When his foot is in the right spot, he is able to slowly stand up out of a slouched position ... I suction and all is well.

Sometimes he lasts a few minutes, other times he can stand for ten or fifteen. He looks awkward and uncomfortable, but he assures me he is fine. I sometimes sit on the floor beside his left leg and hold his foot with my hands.

When Mike told me many months ago that when he can't stand anymore, he will probably decline quickly, because that's what naturally happens when people stop standing, I became as determined as he is. If he hasn't stood in a while, I'll say, "Mike, do you want to stand?" He gives me a smile and a little nod and away we go. But I know my Mike, and I think when he is unable to stand, he'll happily sit and keep fighting. He's a fighter, like those Montreal Canadiens, and there is no giving up.

Montreal and New York play again later today. Mike will be watching and cheering for his team the Canadiens. He is hopeful ...

"Never, never, never give up."

Winston Churchill

The Girl From Agassiz—June 7, 2014

I have some friends I have never met … modern technology makes it possible. I heard from one of those friends this week; she had bad news. It's funny, because she was really on my mind. We hadn't communicated in a long time, but there she was all of a sudden, on my mind. I meant to email her, but she beat me to it.

I first heard from Sharon in an email a couple of years ago. She introduced herself as the chiropractor patient of friends of ours: Darren and his wife Tracey. Sharon told me that her husband had recently been diagnosed with ALS and that she had been reading my blog. We communicated back and forth for a while. We shared our stories and, because Mike was further along in the illness, I was able to answer some questions and give her a little advice.

I remember telling her to get a jump on the home care situation as we had some major issues getting home care and then getting consistent caregivers.

Anyway, after over a year, I heard from Sharon the other day. She reminded me who she was, "The girl from Agassiz … Darren is my Chiropractor." I appreciate reminders, but this time it wasn't necessary. I remembered those things and that her husband's name was Peter (same as my brother-in-law) and that they have three children. She was heavy on my heart just a couple of weeks ago … I definitely remembered her.

Sharon went on to say, "Peter went to be with his Saviour on September 13, 2013 after a brief stay in hospice."

What! I couldn't believe it. He was only diagnosed in May, 2012. She said that when she feels brave, she reads my blog and finds encouragement from it. She said she feels part of me and Mike somehow, as "I see the progression and hear the hurt in your writings." She continued, "The battle belongs to the Lord. I asked God this morning, 'Why, why?' And I am waiting patiently for His response. But each day through my sorrow, I know that He loves me and my beautiful children." And she closed by saying she is praying for us.

I got back to her right away with our condolences and a bunch of questions and she graciously answered them all. She told me the whole story and I cried like a baby. She explained that they couldn't get the home care support they needed. She said that one person would come when two were necessary. She said that she fought hard to get the second person and it finally was okayed, but because of a staff shortage, they often were left with one caregiver or no caregiver, and she couldn't do it on her own. When the social worker suggested that Peter go into hospice, because they would have constant care, they reluctantly agreed. It sounded like they didn't really have a choice.

Sharon says, "I called the kids and they came and we gathered around Peter as he said to us it's a good house, it's been a good time here, kids. Of course, it was a very, very sad time as Peter and I rolled away in the ambulance and had to say goodbye to his house of twenty-two years. It was probably one of the most emotional times in the journey."

She said that Peter's health was good before he went into hospice. He was still breathing well and talking, but as soon as they left their home, his health drastically declined over the course of four days. And regarding that fourth day in hospice,

Sharon said, "The day went quick with family in and out saying their goodbyes. At around 5:00 p.m., it was me and the kids and I gently woke Peter and asked if he was ready to go home to meet Jesus … he opened his eyes, looked at me and said, 'Yes.' I said 'It is okay to go, my sweet Peter, the kids and I release you … no need to fight. We love you.' Shortly thereafter, he took his last breath. It is a heart-wrenching experience. I can't begin to explain the agony of it all."

I can't begin to comprehend the agony of it all, but I can relate to the difficulties of getting proper home care support. Mike and I waited too long to request home care (because that's the way we are), and then when we did request it, it took a long time to even get our case manager over—a nurse from Fraser Health. I remember it was August 2012 and we couldn't get an appointment until October and then it took another few months to get systems in place and actually get the home care support started. Our extremely overworked case manager had to take time off and then lost our paper work. The occupational therapists had to evaluate the environment to make sure it was safe for the home care people for WCB insurance purposes. We had to get lifts in place and there was a concern about the limited space in the bathroom and the quarter-inch lip to get into the shower.

I'm a very calm person, which can be a bit of a detriment. I was having a breakdown on the inside and all was calm and peaceful on the outside, so it looked like I was perfectly fine. When I think back, it's like, "How could I be fine?" But there came a day when I just wasn't okay and I couldn't cope any longer. Still pretty calm on the outside, but close to the edge on the inside, I called Nathan and I called the occupational therapist who I had gotten to know well and knew she would help. They both came over and realized I wasn't okay and the home care delay came to an abrupt end.

My exhaustion didn't end there, though. It took months of training people ... countless people. I kept calling and saying we have to have consistency ... it's imperative! I would remind them that Mike couldn't talk; he was unable to tell the caregiver what he wanted and what to do next. It got to the point where I told them if they were sending a new person, not to bother. It was more work than if I took care of Mike myself. Slowly but surely things started to come together. I called all the time ... I was relentless!

Without proper home care support, managing this illness is impossible. Even with the excellent care we have worked so hard to establish and the support of family, this job is still too big for me, sometimes. It's an extremely important assignment that brings me so much joy, but often overwhelms me. All I can do is take one day at a time and rely on God who is bigger than it all!

When Sharon shared her story with me, I was crushed. I am so sad and at first I was angry at the system that had failed her and her husband. But ultimately, God is in control. He decides when we come and when we go and it was Peter's time to go. I grieve for Sharon and her kids, but rejoice for Peter who is now free from ALS and in the presence of the Lord.

The system will fail us, people will fail us, our bodies will fail us, but God will never fail us!

"So if you are suffering in a manner that pleases God, keep on doing what is right, and trust your lives to the God who created you, for He will never fail you."
I Peter 4:19 NLT

With the news of Peter's passing, that blend of sorrow and joy I have spoken of before has hit an all-time high, or should I say low?

P.S. Mike's caregivers are exceptional! They have become like family … we are so grateful for them!

~ ~ ~ ~ ~ ~ ~

"Heavenly rest will be so refreshing that we will never feel that exhaustion of mind and body we so frequently experience now. I'm really looking forward to that."
Billy Graham

Chapter 17
Challenger Deep

I was learning to let go of Mike long before ALS. Shortly after we got married, I realized that Mike couldn't meet all my needs and I doubted he could fulfill most of my dreams.

Those first few years of marriage were very lonely for me. While Mike went to school in the day and to work at night, I changed a lot of diapers and second-guessed a lot of things. I remember thinking, where is he and why isn't he with me?

But Mike did the right thing ... he had to do what he did for his family, and God had to do what He did in my heart. It's a painful process, but what God wanted to do was teach me to let go of the expectations I had of my husband and put all my expectations in God. He wanted me to look to Him to meet my needs and fulfill all my dreams, and not put those impossible demands on Mike.

It was hard to obey right away; a slow process for sure. But the more I went to God to meet my needs and to be number one to me, the better off Mike and I both were.

Even though we got married because I was pregnant, we were really in love. We have had our share of rough patches for sure, but mostly it's been a deep, passionate, very compatible, and very enduring love. After ten and twenty years, I still sometimes had butterflies in my stomach when Mike pulled up in the driveway.

This ALS journey and all of its challenges have taken our love to an even deeper level ... deep like the deepest depths of the ocean deep, like the Mariana Trench. Mariana Trench is located in the Western Pacific Ocean, south of Japan, just east of the fourteen Mariana Islands near Guam. The very deepest place in Mariana Trench is called "Challenger Deep," located in the southern end of Mariana Trench. Challenger Deep is the deepest known part of the world's ocean at the depth of 36,201 feet.

Sounds like any great, deep love ... challenger deep!

Go West Young Man—June 22, 2014

Mike moved from Ontario to BC in 1985. He and his best friend, Vinroy, hopped on a bus and made the journey as far west as it went. It was for the adventure mostly, but Mike always said he had to come to BC to meet the girl of his dreams ... he said he followed his heart half way across the country to find me.

Vinroy stayed for about two weeks and when his money ran out, he returned home. Mike's money ran out as well, but he stayed and signed up for the army.

While he waited for the summer session to start, he found a cozy spot in a lovely bush on Royal Avenue in New Westminster. We would drive by when our children were little and Mike would say, "Look kids, that's where I lived when I first moved to BC." And they would point and say, "In that big building right there?" and he would point and say, "No, in that bush over there."

Mike had been in the reserves in Ontario and decided to sign up when he got to BC. He joined The Royal Westminster Regiment and that's where he met fellow "Westie": Bob. Funny thing, Nathan became a Westie too and, funnier thing, Nathan had the same commanding officer Mike had had twenty-five years earlier.

Anyway, Bob became Mike's first BC buddy and when their time in the reserves came to an end, Bob invited Mike to move to his hometown, Maple Ridge. This is where Mike eventually met his true love—ME!

Mike and Bob first lived with a few other guys in an old run-down house in town on Macintosh Street. They each kicked in eighty dollars a month to cover the rent.

From there they moved to the "Shack"—five guys and a cat named "Mow" (rhymes with "wow"). Poor Mow could have done better on his own. We were always surprised that cat kept coming back. Those guys never fed Mow, so he was a great little hunter and always appreciated when one of the female visitors would bring treats or a can of cat food. Rent at the Shack was eighty bucks each as well. The Shack is where Mike and I first met.

After the Shack was torn down, Mike and Bob moved to a small apartment over a corner store in Port Coquitlam. It was just the two of them ... no cat and I'm sure rent was more than eighty dollars.

Mike and Bob were good friends for a long time but eventually lost contact. To Mike's surprise, he received a Facebook message from Bob the other day. Bob said he was so sad to hear through a mutual friend that Mike wasn't well. And said he would love to get together some time.

Mike's reply: "Hey Bob, It's good to hear from you. I hope you have been enjoying a good life. You will have to fill me in with the details. As you have heard, I am not doing so well. I have ALS (Lou Gehrig's Disease) ... I've had it for the past four years. They give you three to five years to live, so you can do the math. I am okay with my situation—I have had so many good memories, including the ones I have with you. Everyone has to go sometime ... the trick is to make sure you pack as many good memories in as possible and I think I have done that. Also, I have a strong faith in God and look forward to going to Heaven. Anyway, let me know how you have been doing. Mike."

"My Father's house has many rooms; if that were not so, would I have told you that I am going there to prepare a place for you? And if I go and prepare a place for you, I will come back and take you to be with me that you also may be where I am. You know the way to the place where I am going."
John 14:2-4

~ ~ ~ ~ ~ ~ ~

Bob later messaged me and asked if he could come and visit Mike. I knew Mike wouldn't be crazy about the idea, but of course, I relayed the message anyway. Mike told me he would like to see Bob, but he didn't want Bob to see him. Mike hasn't really wanted anyone from his life pre-ALS to see him now, except family and the friends he was close to at the time of his diagnosis. People get emotional and then Mike gets emotional and he doesn't like it, plus he wants to be remembered the way he was.

I understand, but I think that those excluded from seeing Mike, and from knowing him now are really missing out on something extraordinary.

I feel so blessed to know both Mikes ... pre-ALS Mike is long gone ... someone I miss with tremendous grief. Sometimes I see the old Mike come through the new Mike and for a split second, he's back!

The new Mike is quite exceptional. Spending time with him puts you in touch with something so much bigger than yourself ... you know God is so close! The old Mike answered all my dumb questions and he took care of me. He also joked all the time, which sometimes annoyed me. I'd say, "Mike, just be serious for a minute." But I'd give anything now to spend one day with that jokester. He was serious sometimes too, but I loved how he wanted to make me laugh. The new Mike has let go of the jokes, but still makes me laugh. He has let go of everything and possesses a perfect peace ... he is somewhere between here and heaven.

Our ALS journey has taken our love to a depth it never would have known otherwise and I can't decide if I'd go back if I could.

We still have sex, but I haven't been touched, kissed, hugged, or held by Mike for as long as I can remember and I miss that so much. The old Mike knew just what to do and say to take my breath away; this Mike speaks to me with his eyes and the intimacy is still great—even greater!

Keep Looking Up—July 8, 2014

Madison pointed it out to me when the three of us were out for a walk one day. She said she thought it was weird that I have a fear of flying, but I'm fascinated with airplanes ... every time one flies over, I look up.

I'm actually not fascinated with the plane itself—I don't care about it on the ground—it's more about the machine in the sky. Madison was right; it is kind of weird. But to me, it's just natural ... I have looked up for as long as I can remember and have wondered why most people don't.

We live about 50K away from the Vancouver International Airport, so we aren't that close. It's not like the planes are loud, but still you can hear them, so I look up. Sometimes, I comment. I might say something about its colour or size or if it's flying really high or low, etc. Sometimes, I'll pop a wheelie with Mike's wheelchair so he can see too. And on a nice day or evening, I often say something like, "How wonderful it is to be flying into Vancouver on a day like today." Because, of course, Vancouver is beautiful ... from the sky and the ground!

My dad looks up too. I've really noticed it lately at Nathan's Ultimate Frisbee games ... he and I are looking up while everyone else has their eyes on the game. My dad knows planes ... he flew planes. He had a licence to fly at one time and has always had an interest in planes. While everyone else is watching the Frisbee game, he and I discuss where that one might be coming from and the airline and he always knows what kind of plane it is.

I don't really know why I have to look up when one flies over; but it's like I can't not look up. Regardless, looking up when a plane flies by has caused me to look up thousands of times and looking up is a good thing.

I think the sky is a great reminder of how small we are and how big God is. It's huge and it's uncluttered, unlike some of our spaces, so it helps clear the mind and make troubles disappear for a while. The sky is also in the direction of heaven and they say it's good to look where you are going, not where you have been.

Because of Mike's neck weakness, the physiotherapist from GF Strong recently came and fitted Mike for a neck brace. Mike wasn't crazy about the idea, but I insisted. I told him that transfers would be easier and when he stands, he wouldn't have to work so hard to lift his head up and keep his head up. I also told him van rides would be more enjoyable. Poor Mike is like a bobble head in the van when we go anywhere and I drive super slow and avoid as many bumps as possible ... train tracks are the worst.

Anyway, Mike isn't crazy about his new neck brace. He feels a little suffocated, so he hasn't worn it very much. He did wear it when he and I drove out to Mill Lake in Abbotsford a couple of weeks ago to surprise Neil and Donna at the ALS Walk there (the week before, our "I Like Mike" team participated in the ALS Walk in Port Coquitlam).

We laughed a lot on the way to Mill Lake, because I was asking Mike questions about getting there and with his sunglasses on and his neck brace on, it was almost impossible for him to communicate with me. I couldn't see his eyes and he couldn't nod his head yes or no. Looking at him through the rearview mirror I'd say, "Smile if I exit here ... smile if I turn left here." Trying not to smile made Mike smile more, so needless to say we got a little lost, but we had fun.

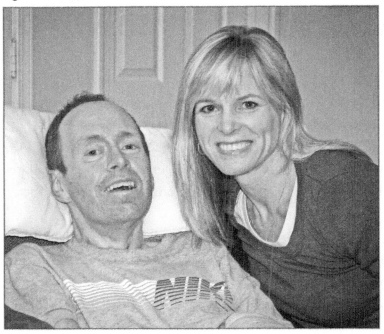

Mike and Nadine
Photo Credit: Ashley Wadhwani

I have never been more in awe of Mike's determination as I am now when I watch him lift his head. When we get him standing up and leaning against his chair, it takes all his might to lift his head. Once it's there, he smiles. Usually, it falls back a little and then he's looking up ... and smiling. Sometimes I help him lift his head and sometimes I hold his head for him, but I also like to hold his feet and support his ankles when he stands, so this can be a bit of a challenge.

Last week when Pat was here, she held Mike's head and I held his feet. Elanna and Madison and whoever else might be around also help sometimes with this juggling act … it's team work at its best!

All I can say is, "Mike, you blow me away! Keep looking up!"

On Track—July 24, 2014

Mike's sister Moira and her husband Mike were here for a visit a few weeks ago. They came a day before Mike's sister Pat got here and left a few days before she did.

Moira isn't a fan of flying and, of course, I can relate. I think her aversion to flying is even stronger than mine. When I heard they were taking the train back home to Toronto, I thought, "What a great idea!"

I would love to take a train across the country. Mike and I had often spoken of doing that together someday. Not only would it be a great way to see the spectacular scenery of each province, but trains travel on the ground (so there's no fear of falling out of the sky like there is in a plane).

This is Mike's message to Moira about a week after they left:

"So I guess you are home by now. Most people taking the train will say the Rocky Mountain portion is enjoyable and that the Prairies are boring because they contain only vast amounts of tall wheat fields that are bland to the eye. I read a book years ago called *Who Has Seen the Wind* by W.O. Mitchell. The last chapter gives a description of the old grandma who is wheelchair bound and sits all day staring out the window at the wheat blowing in the wind. To all around her, people see what appears to be a demented old lady staring into space, but Mitchell's description gives the reader a different outlook on what she sees."

Moira's reply back:

"We just got in this afternoon as our train was five hours behind schedule due to a freight train that had problems ahead. Many times we stopped to allow for freight to pass, as they get priority. No problem for us, as we just sat up in the glass top area watching the scenery and talking with some of the train passengers who were very friendly.

"Although the Prairies were not as spectacular as the Rocky Mountains, they had their own beauty, and we enjoyed watching all of it, including the forest and lake areas after that. We were allowed to get off the train occasionally in small towns along the way for some fresh air and a stretch while the train was serviced, and if you have ever seen the show *Corner Gas*, well, it reminded me of that, with the size of the towns.

"The train was only really rocky one night; the rest of it was normal old-fashioned train rocking, just like the olden days. You felt as though you had been on a train from the 1950s, especially with some of the original bunks and refurbished end of the train lounge car with a cigar/beer table, original redone lounge chairs and decor. It was like that same place on the train in the movie *Double Indemnity* with Fred MacMurray and Barbara Stanwyck, where he steps out the back door for a smoke."

The following is a poem written by our niece Michaela for a school writing assignment:

My uncle is a train.
Always staying on track.
Determined, motivated and knows where it's going.
The outside is made of hard, strong metal
Yet inside is cozy and inviting.
The inside has chairs lined in perfect rows
Which look hard
But once you sit and stay awhile
You realize they have the softest cushions in the world.
In the front, the engineer shovels coal into the fire.
He doesn't stop to take a break or get tired.
Instead he pushes to the limit
In order to keep things running smoothly.
Sometimes the train needs some helpers
And sometimes it can go on its own.
But one thing is certain,
Nothing can stop it.

Free Parking—July 31, 2014

Last week on Wednesday when I took Mike to his bath appointment at the hospital, there was no parking in the free, ten-minute drop-off zone in front of the building where we usually park, so I drove around to the back. We have parked in the back a few times before, but not only is it all pay parking, there is only one wheelchair spot. Thankfully, the one wheelchair parking spot was available and for the sake of the five or ten minutes it takes me to drop Mike off, I wasn't going to worry about paying for parking.

As I was getting Mike out of the van, I could see a couple who looked a little lost walking toward us. They were a beautiful older Indo-Canadian couple in brightly coloured clothing, each walking with a cane. The man came right up to the van and asked if I knew where he could pay for parking. His accent was lovely, but his English a little rough, so there was some confusion when he also showed me the map of where in the hospital they had to go.

I pointed him in the direction of the entrance where the parking machine is and I told him we were going that way and I would help him. He and his wife started walking toward the entrance while I got Mike out of the van. We caught up to them and went in together and I showed him the parking machine. He told me his parking stall number and I punched it in along with the amount of time he wanted. I told him it was six dollars and he pulled out a bunch of change from his pocket. He had a Toonie and two Loonies and a bunch of dimes, so I took the three bigger coins out of his hand and grabbed two Loonies of my own and put the money in and gave him his ticket. He wasn't about to accept my money and insisted I take all of his dimes. He showed me his map again of where he and his wife had to go, so we walked them to the elevator and I explained the rest to him. They thanked us very much and we parted ways.

Yesterday, when I picked Mike up from his bath appointment, we passed a man in the hall talking to medical personnel. I told Mike it looked like the man from last week and continued to our vehicle parked in the free, drop-off zone in the front of the building. As I was wheeling Mike backwards up the ramp into the van, the tall, well-dressed man with a bright blue turban appeared. He tapped his hand on the outside of one thigh a few times and with a big smile said his wife had had her leg surgery and it went well. I said that was great and told him we were happy to hear it. He said, "Do you remember me?"

I said we did; Mike nodded.

He pointed to Mike and said, "What about him?"

I told the man Mike was ill and that he probably wasn't going to get better.

The man came closer and with his finger pointing up, he said, "God is supreme!"

Mike and I nodded in agreement. He said it again and then told us if we pray every morning and every night, everything would be alright. We nodded in agreement and the man said goodbye and walked away.

As we drove off, I got a little choked up and glanced at Mike in the rearview mirror. He was already smiling at me—I smiled back and thought how God is very mysterious, but He keeps things simple at the same time.

His Brains, My Biceps—August 4, 2014

The following is the start of a blog post I never finished from a few months ago … it's a little dark. I'm okay now … things have a way of turning around.

"I've been procrastinating for a while. I don't want to write this blog post, because everyone will know that I'm not as strong as I look; I'm not as strong as everyone thinks I am. I'm weak and thankfully God is strong and that's the only reason I am where I am. I have definitely imagined myself in other places, but by God's grace, I'm in this place … I'm in the palm of His hand.

"I just thought I was dealing with a little bit of mental fatigue, but it's more than that. I call myself crazy sometimes, but my mind is just a little mixed up. I stare at the three toothbrushes and can't decide which one is mine. I know it's purple, but sometimes it takes me a while to determine which one is purple … I think I'm losing it. It's a bunch of stuff: fatigue, burn out, maybe depression. It's the first time in my life I have ever thought, 'What's the point?'"

There was more, but you get the drift. Those feelings didn't last that long—about two months. But on a regular basis, I am mentally drained … I forget stuff all the time and I get a little mixed up. I often tell Mike that between the two of us, we make one great person … with his brains and my biceps (and the rest of my body), we really function well. Anyway, I didn't tell anyone I definitely wasn't functioning well during those couple of months, but my sister kept asking if I was okay and Erin was encouraging me to get away.

I kept saying I was fine and I told Erin I'd go away for a day or two when Aunt Pat came … that was around April or the beginning of May. Pat was coming sometime in June. When she confirmed she was coming the last weekend in June, I asked Nathan to stay overnight on the Saturday of that weekend. I knew between our two sisters and the kids and Mike's regular home care support people, he would be well taken care of … even still, it's really hard to leave him.

When I heard the workshop I was interested in attending was happening that weekend, I signed up. It was called "InspireABook"—a two-day intensive for potential authors wanting to gain knowledge about writing and publishing a book. I was really excited about the workshop, but not about leaving Mike.

Leaving Mike for a whole day or more is agony, but not having a day away every once in a while is painful too. It's the greatest internal tug of war I'm sure I'll ever know.

I'm going away again tomorrow for a couple of days. Erin is having hip replacement surgery tomorrow, so of course, I will be with her for the day and I will spend the night with her at the UBC Hospital. Pat and Aileen are coming to help and with the help of my family too, Mike and Erin will both be well cared for!

The InspireABook workshop was great ... and exhausting. At the end of the first day, Julie, author and founder and publisher of Influence Publishing (CEO), who led the workshop took me aside and told me she wanted to publish my book and handed me some paper work—a contract. She told me to read it over with Mike and she said she was really excited about my book.

After deciding to write a book and after researching everything I could about publishing, I was a little overwhelmed and then a friend told me about Influence Publishing, a company based here in Vancouver. I looked into it and thought it was perfect for me. I'd sent Julie a book proposal about a month before the workshop. I kept thinking, "This is really dumb ... or maybe it's pretty good ..." I had no idea. Anyway, she liked it and I have embarked on something really exciting ... telling Mike's story in a book ... our story.

What else is exciting is Erin's new hip. The end of a long journey and the beginning of something great. And that's a whole other story ...

"The wind really was boisterous and the waves really were high, but Peter didn't see them at first. He didn't consider

*them at all; he simply recognized his Lord, stepped out
in recognition of Him, and 'walked on the water' ... You
do not know when His voice will come to you, but whenever the realization of God comes, even in the faintest way
imaginable, be determined to recklessly abandon yourself,
surrendering everything to Him. It is only through aban-
donment of yourself and your circumstances that you will
recognize Him."*
Oswald Chambers

Pouring Buckets—August 22, 2014

They say when it rains it pours and that's exactly what's been
happening around here lately. It's been pouring buckets for the
last few weeks, but before I say anything about the Ice Bucket
Craze for ALS, I'm going to back things up to last Saturday.

I was spending a lot of time with Erin who was recovering
from her hip replacement surgery, but I had come home for
a little while to see Mike ... I was so thankful Aileen and Pat
were here for the week making it possible for me to go back
and forth.

I had just left the house and was heading back to Erin's when I
got a call from my mom. I had left my parents a message earlier
asking if they had heard back from the doctor regarding my
dad's recent blood test results.

My dad had been to the doctor a few days before at the
prompting of some friends who thought his skin looked a
little yellow. I noticed his colour was off too, kind of like a
spray tan gone bad. My dad has never had a spray tan—he's
probably never heard of a spray tan, so maybe I should have
said something.

Anyway, my mom returned my call to tell me they had heard back from the doctor about the blood work and that the doctor sent my dad straight to the hospital, because something wasn't right and they wanted to do more tests.

So then I found myself at the 7-Eleven by the hospital picking up snacks and a puzzle book for my dad ... I felt like I was dreaming. Only a half an hour earlier, I was suctioning the back of Mike's throat and a few hours before that, I was doing Erin's laundry and helping her with her mobility exercises, and a week before that I was sitting beside my dad out in the backyard with the rest of the family listening to him recall stories from his all-time favourite trip to Paraguay.

My dad has lots of interesting and exciting stories about his travels. I tell him he should write a book. He says he will when he retires from his missionary work ... but he also says he's never going to retire.

If you ask him about this particular trip to Paraguay, he reminds you again it is his very favourite. It was a trip to connect with his parents' past and learn about the history of his ancestors and meet relatives he never knew.

His parents, along with a large Mennonite community from Manitoba, followed their hopes and dreams to a place they were told was a land of milk and honey. This was in the late 1920s before my dad was born.

The milk and honey turned out to be Typhoid Fever and many members of the group died, including my dad's aunt and sister. My grandmother was so devastated and very sick herself, she just wanted to go home. So back to Manitoba they went and started again from scratch.

My dad's eyes light up when he talks about travelling on

the beautiful Paraguay River and visiting the land his parents tried to build a life on. He tells you about seeing the spot his baby sister was laid to rest, along with his aunt, and about the connections he made with the relatives still there.

The first thought that came to my mind when I heard my dad was in the hospital was this visit in the backyard the week prior and the feeling I got while I listened to this story I have heard many times before ... the feeling was a lovely, peaceful, feeling. I just relaxed and listened and loved how excited he was to tell about it again ... and, yes, I wondered about his weird tan.

The weird tan was a symptom and the CT scan revealed a tumour near his pancreas and a biopsy revealed cancer. Wow, it was quite a blow for sure and, like they say, when it rains it pours and sometimes, it pours buckets ... even during the sunniest month of the year.

While we waited for test results to see if the cancer had spread, we of course prayed and hoped for the best. While we prayed and hoped for the best, another prayer was being answered.

This is what I said about the recent ALS fundraiser phenomenon in an article I wrote for *iVillage*, a Corus Entertainment property and women's lifestyle website based in Toronto.

"Recently, Lou Gehrig's disease has been in the spotlight with the viral 'Ice Bucket Challenge' fundraiser—a movement to raise awareness and funds for ALS.

"I've been watching from the sidelines and feel like I'm cheering the underdog on to victory. In a matter of a few weeks, ALS quickly inundated our news feeds. Pro athletes, musicians, politicians, big name celebrities, and others are getting in on it, including Oprah and Bill Gates ...

"ALS gets some much-needed and well-deserved attention and I think that's great. Finally people are hearing about it, awareness and funds are being raised, and our hope for a cure has been renewed. And it puts a smile on my husband's face when he hears, 'This one's for you.'"

I was honoured to be asked by Russell, an editor of *iVillage* to give my opinion on the Ice Bucket Challenge. He said he had come across my blog and was interested in my writing and our lives with ALS. The article was well received and shared on OWN Oprah Winfrey Network: Canada, W Network, and CNT Network Facebook pages, along with many others.

So, needless to say, it's been pouring buckets ... literally. And this is where we are at today: Erin is recovering well from her hip surgery and she is almost off the pain medication that has taken a bit of a toll on her stomach. It looks like my dad's cancer is contained and he will have surgery as soon as possible to remove the tumour. And regarding the Ice Bucket Challenge, millions of dollars have been raised and perhaps even better than that, more people are aware of this devastating disease.

Mike's response spelled out in a quiet whisper: "i-s-n-t t-h-i-s g-r-e-a-t."

~ ~ ~ ~ ~ ~ ~

Russell got back to me after he read my article and said something like, "I really like this, this and this, but can you tell us about a day in your life? Give us the straight goods ... be real."

So I revised the article and included the following, "Mike specialized in psychiatric nursing and he was well respected in his field. Such a smart, well educated, competent man, and now his wife wipes his butt and other people shower him. He takes food through a feeding tube and chokes on a little bit of saliva."

The edited paragraph said, "Mike specialized in psychiatric nursing but now he needs a nurse. He needs help in the bathroom, takes food through a feeding tube, and can't stand on his own."

I just smiled, because I thought perhaps what I wrote was a little too "real" for the world just getting to know about ALS.

Ice Bucket List—August 28, 2014—by Mike Sands

In the Christmas movie *Elf*, Santa Claus is seen stranded in Central Park, New York. The motor on his sleigh breaks down and Buddy the elf attempts to fix it. As Buddy works on the sleigh, Santa explains to Buddy that in the good old days he would never have this problem, because his sleigh was powered by the spirit of Christmas.

Buddy's girlfriend convinces a crowd to join her in singing Christmas carols. The group's singing is broadcasted nationwide and soon everyone is singing, which raises the spirit of Christmas to new heights. Santa's sleigh is soon seen soaring in the sky.

I had my first symptoms of ALS four years ago this month. Over the past four years, I have lost the ability to walk, talk, move most of my body, and swallow properly; in essence, every muscle in my body has stopped working or is on its way to that result.

It's understandable for anyone in these circumstances to be in low spirits. As I experience my body deteriorating on a daily basis, I look for things to raise my spirits, and the recent ALS Ice Bucket Challenge has done this. The money raised is great, but what's even more important is that the challenge is a sign that society is in our corner, ready to fight this disease with us arm in arm.

Right now with my elevated spirits, I think I could guide Santa's sleigh clear around the world.

~ ~ ~ ~ ~ ~ ~

> It took Mike a few days to write this blog post, even though he knew exactly what he wanted to say. With his head mouse, Mike typed one letter at a time on his communication device, the DynaVox, and I wrote it out for him on the blog. His neck muscles don't last long, so his window of time to write is very limited. We are in the process of getting something called "eye gaze," where you just have to use your eyes to move the cursor.

For Better or Worse—September 19, 2014

The day Mike was diagnosed with ALS, he told us he didn't want a tracheal tube to help him breathe when the illness progresses to that point. A tracheal tube is invasive mechanical ventilation that requires a tracheostomy for placement of a tube into the windpipe to deliver air directly into the lungs. It's an excellent solution for some people who choose to go that route, but Mike has long ago made up his mind not to go that route. Every once in a while throughout this journey, I have asked Mike if he still feels the same way about this "trach" topic and without hesitation, he responds, "Yes." It's Mike's life and as much as I want him to be with me for as long as possible, I would never try to talk him into a tracheal tube. He says it will just prolong the inevitable and he says he would rather be doing cartwheels in heaven than be stuck here, completely paralyzed, non-verbal, and breathing through a tube. I don't blame him ... I think I'd feel the same way.

Sometimes I watch Mike breathe; at night mostly when he sleeps. I stare at his chest to see it rise and fall, and I delight in the small movement and in the odd deep breath. Of course, the inability to breathe is what makes this illness fatal, so even though Mike is almost fully paralyzed, those deep breaths give me hope; there's still time.

This summer, Mike was listed as "palliative." While anyone diagnosed with a terminal illness is considered palliative, when Mike was *listed* as palliative, I was left with a lump in my throat for days. When you hear "palliative" you think, "dying" and while Mike *is* dying of ALS, we've never really thought of it as *dying* of ALS, but instead, "*living* with ALS."

Palliative care is specialized medical care for people with serious/incurable illness. The focus of palliative care is to keep the patient comfortable. Doctors and nurses work with the existing medical team to provide an extra layer of support. The goal is a better quality of life.

When Mike was listed as palliative, we were told that doctors and nurses would come to our house to see us and offer support as needed. We were also told that Mike would start getting medication for free and perhaps even home care for free and other "perks." We thought, "Wow, membership has its privileges." Had we known these things, perhaps we would have signed up earlier.

Sure enough, we have had visits from the community palliative nurses and someone from the Provincial Respiratory Outreach Program who brought a non-invasive breathing machine called a BiPAP and a back-up suction machine. The palliative doctor came for a visit as well. She prescribed Mike a liquid compound medication for his excessive secretions, which goes in his tube. It has helped, but lately, I must say the faucet has been running again.

Even though Mike has recently been listed as palliative, we are not discouraged and even though Mike has made a firm decision regarding invasive breathing apparatus, we as a family are not discouraged ... we make the best of this life with ALS however long or short it is ... we are at peace ... we actually feel extremely blessed.

This world is in a sorry state of affairs. ALS is just a drop in the bucket when it comes to trials and tribulation. So many people on this planet are experiencing far worse. I can't watch the news very often, it's just far too upsetting. Sometimes I say, "I should have watched that Seinfeld rerun again instead of the news." And we drag ourselves to bed feeling terrible for others and grateful to be us.

Ah, life ... no one warned it was going to be so unfair, but no one promised it was going to be wonderful either, and isn't it both? Don't we need to take the bad with the good? Mike and I embrace both, because without the one, we wouldn't have the other.

When we take our beloved partner in marriage, we take them "for better or worse." We accept their faults for our favourite things about them. It's a package deal ... kind of like life! We accept the faults and our favourite things about it, and, like Mike would say, "It's good to be alive!"

Other news around here:

- Teachers are no longer on strike here in BC, so Erin is very happy to be back to work! And she continues to recover well from her hip-replacement surgery.
- Leah starts Kindergarten! Following in her dad's footsteps (and aunts' and cousins'), she is going into French Immersion … *très bien*!
- I have gone back to school as well, along with Madison. We are taking the SETA (Special Education Teacher Assistant) course. I've been interested in this program for a long time and am so thrilled to be taking it now with Madison! This has been a big step for me, because not only is it a challenge with my time, it also kind of breaks my heart to "move forward" when I just really want to stay "here" with Mike.
- My dad continues to wait for a surgery date to remove his cancerous tumour and is upset because he says had he known he would have to wait this long, he would have followed through with his plans to go to Malawi. He has a building project going on there, plus he has more wells to drill. He says he's got to get back—there's a lot more work to do. I'm sure he'll be back before we know it. The plan is for Nathan to accompany him next time.
- The Ice Bucket challenge has come and gone, but lingers on around here … just the other day we had a surprise video from Vinroy, Mike's best buddy from Toronto whom he hasn't seen in years and who I just mentioned in my recent post, "Go West Young Man." Mike and I were both in tears watching the heartwarming video. Just before Vinroy has the freezing cold bucket of ice water dumped on his head,

he says, "This one's for you Mike. If it wasn't for you, I wouldn't be here … you know what I mean." Mike saved Vinroy from drowning when they were teenagers. Mike has actually saved a few people from drowning.

- Also, while the Bucket Challenge was going strong, Jerrica, a young woman from our community, started a fundraiser for us on Facebook. I first met Jerrica when she organized a fundraiser for Project Wellness at her high school, a few years back. It was a huge success and she kept thanking me for speaking at the event. I had to laugh, because she was doing us the favour, and I kept thanking her. Thank you, Jerrica, once again, and thank you everyone for your very kind and encouraging words and generous Ice Bucket donations!

- I am almost finished writing my book. In order for it to be on shelves in the spring, the manuscript is due next Friday. For weeks I've been saying, "It's almost done!" But there's still a ways to go in tying up loose ends. Everyone has been so patient with me as it's been my primary focus for months. Thanks to Madison for all the salads, sandwiches, muffins, and other meals!

Well, that list of news is a lot of *good* news. I'll go to bed tonight with a happy heart and watch Mike's chest rise and fall, and delight in every breath. And I'll give thanks to God, of course!

One final thing. We have lived here with Elanna and Peter and kids for over two years now (three summers), and they continue to stick by our side "for better or worse." While Michaela and Luke are teenagers and would probably love to have their rec room space, we never hear a complaint. We never hear a complaint about anything from any of them. We are grateful beyond words for their help and support and we couldn't do it without them!

~ ~ ~ ~ ~ ~ ~

Bottom line, our story is a love story. It's about God's awesome and infinite love, the wonderful love of family and friends, and our "Challenger Deep" love for each another.

On April 3, 2014, I wrote in my journal: "This morning while Mike and I were in the bathroom, I talked while he took a "TC." When I dumped the bucket from his commode in the toilet, he laughed a little. I thought he's got to be laughing because this is absolutely crazy. Who would have thunk it on our wedding day that I'd be wiping his butt today?

I said something to him about how crazy it was of us to run away and get married. I asked him, "Is that the craziest thing you have ever done?"

He nodded no.

I said it was the craziest thing I've ever done.

He spelled B—E—S—T.

I said, "It's the BEST thing you have ever done?"

He nodded yes and started crying. I held him and we both cried … and then I finished wiping his butt.

Faith, hope, and love are what we hold on to as we let go … and the greatest of these is love!

ALS With Courage—Our Story in Pictures

More photographs can be viewed on the blog, ALS
With Courage, and on Facebook:
www.alswithcourage.com
www.facebook.com/ALSWithCourage

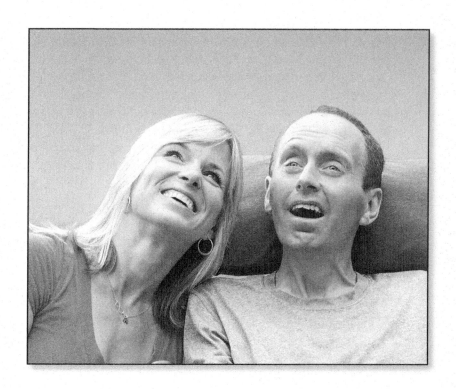

"Keep looking up ... it's the secret of life."
Snoopy

Author Biographies

Nadine Sands has spent many years working as a certified fitness instructor and personal trainer and, along with her husband Michael, has also raised three children. Before Michael's diagnosis with ALS (otherwise known as Lou Gehrig's disease), Nadine and her husband were an active couple who enjoyed various sports, as well as hiking and biking. Nadine was also actively involved in her family's charity, Project Wellness.

When they discovered that Michael had ALS, a terminal illness, Nadine became his full-time, primary caregiver. She 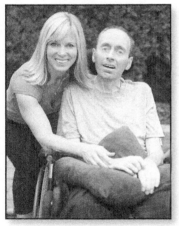 started a blog about their journey as a couple called *ALS With Courage*. She is passionate about sharing her and her husband's inspirational story and raising awareness about ALS.

Mike Sands was born and raised in Scarborough, Ontario. He moved to British Columbia in 1985 at the age of twenty-three and joined the army. Soon after, he moved to Maple Ridge, BC, and met the love of his life, Nadine. Mike and Nadine got married and five years later had their third child to complete their family. During those years, Mike went back to school to become a nurse.

Mike was working two jobs as a registered nurse, specializing in Psychiatric Nursing, when in 2011 he was diagnosed with ALS. Nadine was Mike's primary caregiver and the two resided with Nadine's sister and family in their ground-level basement suite.

Obituary

Michael David Sands (1962-2015)

His glass was always half full. Lessons to be learned from this courageous man: Give thanks in all circumstances. Have faith, be hopeful, and love deeply. Talk is cheap so walk the walk. Be generous. Never give up! And if you don't have a napkin, just wipe your hands on your socks (he always wore knee-highs).

Our beloved Son, Brother, Husband, Father, Granddad, Uncle, Nephew, Cousin, and friend was called home to heaven on Monday, January 5th. His chains are gone—he's been set free! He's doing cartwheels now with Jesus and enjoying steak dinners and fettuccine. Mike battled ALS for four years with brilliance, and when the Lord called him to give up the fight, he humbly obeyed.

A friend says, "Though his earthly body may have 'lost the battle with ALS,' his spirit conquered it tenfold."

Mike will be dearly missed, but his lessons live on forever!

A celebration of the life he left behind and his new life in glory took place on Mike's birthday, January 16 at 3:30 p.m. at Maple Ridge Baptist Church. In lieu of flowers, donations to Project Wellness were greatly appreciated. A memorial well was drilled in Malawi, Africa in Mike's name.

My dearest Michael, I love you to the moon and back compared to an ant ... and far more than that.

Your sweetheart, Nadine

If you want to get on the path to becoming a published author with Influence Publishing please go to www.InfluencePublishing.com

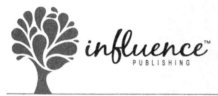

Inspiring books that influence change

More information on our other titles and how to submit your own proposal can be found at www.InfluencePublishing.com

CPSIA information can be obtained at www.ICGtesting.com
Printed in the USA
LVOW04s2309150315

430598LV00007B/46/P